Best wishes,

*Back to Basics*

# *Back to Basics*

A Practical Guide to Healthier Eating and Weight Loss

## April Adams, RD

Books by April
Whiteland, Indiana

Back to Basics
Copyright © 2007 by April Adams

Published by Books by April in 2007

All rights reserved. No part of this book may be used or reproduced in any manner whatsoever without the prior written permission of the publisher, except in the case of brief quotations embodied in critical articles or reviews.

Cover design and all photographs by Mark Matthews

ISBN 978-0-615-17902-5

Printed in the United States of America

10 9 8 7 6 5 4 3 2 1

www.booksbyapril.com

*To Jared,*
my wonderfully supportive husband, for without your countless hours of help, this book would not have been possible.

*To my family and friends,*
who took the time to read the book, gave positive and constructive feedback, and helped take care of my precious kiddos while I wrote.

*To you,*
who have read the book or are about to, thank you for entrusting me to guide you along your weight loss journey. I hope and pray that you will truly be inspired to become a healthier version of you.

# *Contents*

*Getting Started*
1

*Nutrition 101*
11

*Tips*
33

*Wrap-up*
83

*Resources*
85

*About the Author*
108

# Getting Started

In this book you will find:
- ❖ A brief discussion of the basic physiology of weight loss
- ❖ Basic nutrition information
- ❖ A discussion of the sources of calories
- ❖ Tips for increasing physical activity
- ❖ An overview of the Food Pyramid, including the recommended number of servings from each food group and appropriate portion sizes
- ❖ How to design a balanced meal
- ❖ How to calculate your Ideal Body Weight and a discussion of Body Mass Index
- ❖ **A list of practical tips to help you learn to eat healthier and cut unnecessary calories**
- ❖ A week's worth of sample menus
- ❖ A sample meal pattern that will allow you to design your own meals
- ❖ A sample food record evaluation to help you learn how to evaluate your current diet
- ❖ A sample grocery list based on a week's worth of meals

The purpose of this book is to provide practical, down-to-earth tips for how to eat healthier and lose weight. As a Registered Dietitian (RD), I have been approached by family, friends, neighbors, co-workers, and patients seeking advice on weight loss. I've sat at the kitchen table, talked on the phone, emailed, snail-mailed, and sat with patients in my office in an attempt to provide practical, healthy, weight loss tips in a concise way. I cannot count the number of times I've given out the same information over and over and I'm always afraid that I'm leaving out something critical, so I decided to put it all in one place. Now, when someone asks me for advice on weight loss or a healthier diet, I'll be able to refer them here knowing that all of my tips are in one place. In order to make this book as practical as possible, I simply captured what I do or have done in my own everyday diet to save calories and meet nutrient needs. So as you begin to adopt these eating habits, you can know that I've not given you tips that are impossible to maintain because I do them or have done them myself.

If you're wondering why there are some tips that I "have done" (meaning that I no longer or don't always do them), it's because there have been times when I've needed to be more diligent about cutting calories than others (e.g., losing post-baby weight). Once I met my goal weight and began to simply maintain, I discovered that certain tips for cutting calories didn't need to be followed as closely. You may find the same with yourself.

All of the tips in this book are meant to help you learn to eat healthier and cut unnecessary calories, so once you reach your goal weight you should be able to be a bit more lenient. Obviously, if you were to become too lenient and regain some weight, you would simply pick back up some of the tips you stopped doing. I weigh myself regularly and if I happen to notice that I've gained a couple of pounds, then I know to tighten the reins a bit. Weight loss is such a personal system of trial and error. I recommend you start by trying to follow the tips as closely as possible and then give yourself some leeway as you're able.

You'll notice quickly (if you haven't already!) that this book is not academic or deeply scientific; it's just a simple guide with practical tips that you can incorporate into everyday life. This book is NOT meant to provide you with a temporary diet for quick weight loss. Rather, it is meant to teach you how to eat healthier from now on so that you can achieve a healthy weight at a slow, gradual rate and keep it off in the long run. If at all possible, I would prefer that you not concentrate so much on numbers in regards to weight loss. If you look at this as simply learning to eat healthier in order to BE healthier, then if you need to lose weight it will happen. Let go of the stress of constantly thinking about calories, points, fat, carbs, and pounds and retrain your mind to think more about your overall health.

A common theme found throughout the book is that **you should be able to eat ALL foods in moderation.** My philosophy on weight loss is that one should simply learn to make healthier choices and to eat in moderation. I don't believe that there are any "bad foods" you need to always avoid. I've heard that an estimated 90-95% of American dieters regain all of their weight lost on a diet within five years. Is that because overweight Americans are genetically destined to be overweight or that it's practically impossible for them to achieve a healthy weight? I don't believe so. I propose that most dieters are simply choosing the wrong path to weight loss. They're choosing quick-fix methods, like fad diets, shakes, juices, or pills, which promise results without the need for life*long*, life*style* changes. Quick-fix weight loss methods don't work in the long-run, and I hope that after reading this book you will decide to never waste your time or money on them again.

## *Why fad diets don't work*

If you've ever tried a fad diet (and most of us have, unfortunately) think back to some of them. By "fad diet," I mean any sort of restrictive weight loss diet (e.g., Atkins, Sugar Busters, Cabbage Soup, Grapefruit, Zone). Consider the following questions:

- ❖ What fad diets have you tried?
- ❖ How long did you follow them on average?
- ❖ Why aren't you still following them?
- ❖ Why didn't they work?

Fad diets often promise quick weight loss, which is quite appealing. However, they're just too hard to maintain in the long-run. They set you up for failure because they often lead to frustration and an eventual surrender to your old eating habits, which causes you to regain the weight you lost and return to square one. Such yo-yo dieting leaves you worse-off in the long run. **When evaluating a diet, ask yourself this one question: "Can I follow this for the rest of my life?"** If the answer is no, then you will eventually stop following the diet and regain all of the weight you lost. What's the point of going through all of that just to end up back where you started?

This book does not provide you with a temporary diet; rather, with an eating plan, a way of life. Healthy weight loss involves lifelong changes to your diet so that you can maintain it in the long-run. If you think that you're going to follow the latest fad diet for a few weeks or months, then that's how long the weight loss will last — a few weeks or months. As soon as you go back to your old ways, the weight will creep back on.

The truth about long-term weight loss is that there are no magic bullets or quick fixes and if a weight loss product or diet sounds "too good to be true," IT IS. The good news is that you don't have to be a slave to a diet, you don't have to avoid all treats, and you don't have to be hungry in order to achieve your weight loss goal as long as you're willing to lose at a slow, gradual pace.

Think of weight loss in terms of running. Fad diets are like a sprint, whereas healthy weight loss is more like a marathon. Visualize a sprinter. Consider how she starts the race: knelt down in a position that will allow her to shoot off the starting block as quickly as possible. A sprinter musters up all of her energy and gives it all she has for a short distance. There's no possible way that a sprinter could maintain her speed for the length of a marathon; she would burn out within minutes. This is much like a fad dieter. You muster up your enthusiasm and follow the restrictive guidelines as closely as possible, avoiding all treats, until finally, you burn out.

On the other hand, visualize a marathon runner. Consider how he starts the race: standing upright, muscles warm but relaxed, he begins at a slow, gradual pace that will allow him to continue the race until the end, miles away. He must maintain a conserved, yet steady pace so that he won't burn out before he crosses the finish line. This is comparable to healthy weight loss. You must allow yourself to eat all foods in moderation, including treats, so that you can maintain the diet for the rest of your life, and so that you don't burn out and give up. Healthy weight loss is a marathon, not a sprint.

## *Already at a healthy weight?*

You may be completely comfortable with your current weight and simply want to learn how to eat healthier- this book can help you too. Realize that just because your body is at a healthy weight doesn't mean that you provide it with an adequate amount of nutrients so that it functions the best it can. A healthy, balanced diet that provides a variety of nutrients is vital to the thousands of processes that occur in your body every day. A healthy diet can help prevent chronic diseases such as high blood pressure, heart disease, Type 2 diabetes, osteoporosis, and certain cancers.

Also consider that if you have children, their eating habits will strongly reflect yours. Eat healthier in order to be a good role model for them. Children certainly need a healthy diet in order to keep up with the nutrient demands of growth and development. Good childhood nutrition is also important for the prevention of long-term diseases such as those mentioned above. The information in this book is meant for adults, but can certainly be applied to children age 2 and up as well. Realize, however, that portion sizes are smaller for ages 2–8. Check out mypyramid.gov for age-specific recommendations.

## *Want to lose weight?*

You may be at a point in your life where you've tried every fad diet that's crossed your path in a desperate effort to lose weight, or perhaps this is your first attempt. Wherever you are in your weight loss journey, whether you need to lose five pounds or 500, the tips in this book can help. You may find one tip that helps you lose those last few pounds, or you may find several tips that, together, will help you lose many pounds. If you gradually adopt them, you will lose weight at a healthy rate that is right for your body. A healthy rate of weight loss is about 0.5–2 pounds per week. A loss of more than two pounds per week, in most cases, indicates loss of water and lean muscle. Your goal should be to lose fat, not muscle.

As you begin your weight loss journey, please realize that it is very common to hit plateaus where you stop losing for a period of time. Such plateaus can occur without warning after a nice, steady pace of weight loss. This is completely normal. Don't let these plateaus discourage you—keep going. Your body is probably just adjusting to the change in caloric intake and shift in metabolism, and if you stick with the guidelines and follow the tips consistently, you will continue to close in on your goal weight. Again, I prefer that you pay less attention to the number on the scale and more attention to how your clothes fit and how you feel. I realize, however, that the scale is an objective way to measure your success and that it can help you see that you're on the right track. Try to limit weigh-ins to once per week since weight can fluctuate due to fluid shifts, especially for the ladies.

I want so much for you to succeed in reaching a healthy weight because I know how much better you will feel both physically and mentally when you begin to make progress and eventually meet your goal. As you begin, you will be more likely to succeed if you start with a reasonable goal. If you start with unreasonable expectations, then you'll be easily disappointed and more likely to give up. Research has shown that losing just 10% of your current body weight can reduce your risk of health complications associated with being overweight, so use that as a starting point. If you currently weigh 200 pounds, make it your first goal to lose 20 pounds; once you reach 180 pounds, shoot for an 18-pound weight loss, and so on until you reach your ultimate goal.

Take your mind off of short-term weight loss and start thinking about the long-term. Which of the following approaches makes more sense to you? Try a fad diet, lose 10–30 pounds quickly, get burned out, give up, and regain all the weight plus more. Or, take the time to learn to eat healthier, lose weight gradually, and maintain a healthy weight for life. I've counseled many patients seeking weight loss and the majority of them have the same story. They try a fad diet (e.g., Atkins, South Beach, Medifast, Grapefruit, Cabbage Soup) or take an over-the-counter weight loss product (e.g., pills, shakes, juices) for a few weeks to a few months, lose 0 to 30 pounds or so, get burned out, give up, and then make up for lost time and regain 40 pounds. If you're ready to give up dieting, then keep reading and remember that we're doing this together because these tips continue to work for me and others every day.

# Nutrition 101

## Calories In vs. Calories Out

Before we get to the tips, I want to give you some information on the physiology of weight loss and the basics of a healthy diet so that you will better understand why each tip is in here. First, you must understand **that the key to weight loss is simply a net loss of calories**. Weight gain is generally a result of consuming more calories than your body spends. In other words, your weight is a direct result of the amount of calories you put into it (unless you have a medical condition, such as congestive heart failure, that causes your weight to fluctuate due to fluid gains and losses).

Calories are energy for your body much like gas is fuel for a car; your body requires a certain number of calories to work just like your car requires a certain amount of gas to run. The difference is that if you put too much gas in your car, the gas would simply run out of the tank and pour out onto the ground, whereas if you put more calories into your body than it needs, it stores those extra calories as fat. Your body was created to survive so that if faced with a famine or shortage in food supply, you would have the ability to use those fat stores for energy. Fortunately (or unfortunately), in America, most of us have access to an abundance of food, so very few of us would ever need to call upon our fat stores to save us from starvation. So, as we pour in unnecessary calories without burning them in physical activity, our bodies become fatter. **The goal in weight loss, therefore, is to achieve a net loss of calories by consuming fewer calories in the foods we choose and spending more calories in physical activity.**

If you liken the concept of weight loss to a "fat" bank account that you are trying to empty, think of calories as money. The only way to lessen the money in your bank account is to either put less in or take more out. I would suggest both. In other words, you will need to start putting fewer calories into your body and start spending more calories in regular physical activity. It takes a net loss of 3500 calories to lose a pound of fat, whether that net loss is achieved by cutting caloric intake or by increasing calories spent in physical activity. For example, if you were to cut 300 unnecessary calories per day from your diet and spend an extra 200 calories in activity (a total of 500 calories per day), you would lose approximately 1 pound per week (500 calories per day times 7 days per week).

You may be wondering how many calories you should be eating in a day. You may also be thinking that if the key to weight loss is simply a net loss in calories,

# BACK TO BASICS

why not cut way back and follow a very low-calorie diet with 800 or 1000 calories per day? For one, following a very low-calorie diet is a quick-fix weight loss method (a sprint) and one that you cannot maintain long-term. Also, when you go from a high calorie diet, such as 3500 calories or more per day (which you may be consuming now) down to 1000 calories per day, your body assumes that you must be facing a famine and potential starvation, so it lowers your metabolism to conserve energy as long as possible.

Also consider that if you currently consume 3500 calories per day and you cut back to 2500, you will (theoretically) lose 2 pounds per week (a net loss of 1000 calories per day x 7 days per week = 7000 calories, divided by 3500 calories per pound of fat = 2 pounds of fat per week). All you need to do is cut out 500–1000 unnecessary calories from your current diet in order to lose 1–2 pounds per week. That's much less painful than trying to follow an impossibly restrictive low-calorie diet.

## *Calorie Sources*

Before we go any further, let me discuss the three primary sources of calories: carbohydrate, protein, and fat. Our bodies require all of these in order to be healthy and work properly, so removing any of them from the diet is not healthy. Instead, it's important to learn how to balance your diet with the right amounts of each.

**Carbohydrate** is in the form of simple sugars and complex sugars (starches) and provides four calories per gram (4 cals/gram). Carbohydrates are essential to a healthy diet for many reasons, some of which are discussed later. Despite the bad name sugar has been given as a result of the low-carb diet craze, our bodies actually need it to work properly. In fact, the brain uses carbohydrates as its most efficient source of energy (as opposed to protein or fat). If you've ever followed a low-carb/high protein diet, you may have noticed a loss in concentration (not to mention the many other ill effects of that diet), which can be attributed to the lack of glucose (a type of sugar) available to the brain. Foods that contain simple sugars include fruit and fruit juice, milk, yogurt, and of course, cookies, cakes, ice cream, pies, jelly, syrup, candy, regular soda, etc. Complex sugars, or starches, include bread, pasta, cereal, rice, crackers, tortillas, bagels, English muffins, beans, lentils, and certain vegetables (e.g., peas, corn, and potatoes).

Another source of calories is **protein**, which also provides four calories per gram (4 cals/gram). Proteins are also essential to a healthy diet as they provide the building blocks for muscles, bones, skin, and hormones. In addition, they help repair the body's tissues and help the immune system work properly. I don't think I need to convince many of you to eat adequate protein because we Americans tend to eat plenty of it – too much of it actually. Examples of protein-rich foods include meat, fish, poultry, cheese, cottage cheese, eggs, and tofu.

The last main source of calories is **fat**, which provides nine calories per gram (9 cals/gram). Notice that fat provides more calories than carbohydrates and proteins combined. Again, fats are a necessary part of a healthy diet as some of them provide "essential fatty acids" (EFA). One EFA you may have heard of is omega-3 fatty acid. This one has been shown to have anti-inflammatory properties, which is believed to help reduce the risk of heart disease. Fats are also a good source of vitamin E. Examples of fats include oil, butter, margarine, shortening, nuts, seeds, olives, mayonnaise, cream cheese, bacon, regular salad dressing, and sour cream. Good sources of omega-3 fatty acids include fish, especially salmon and tuna; shellfish; flaxseed; and walnuts.

If a product contains 10 grams of fat, 10 grams of carbohydrate, and 10 grams of protein, the fat would provide 90 calories (9 cals/gram), the carbohydrate would provide 40 calories (4 cals/gram) and the protein would provide 40 calories (4 cals/gram) for a grand total of 170 calories. As you may notice, the calories from fat add up the fastest since it contains twice as many calories per gram as carbohydrate and protein.

I certainly don't expect you to memorize all of these numbers. I explained all of that in order to illustrate that **fat is the richest source of calories in our diet, which is why limiting the fat in your diet can help with weight management.** If you currently eat a high-fat diet, lowering your intake of fat is one of the quickest ways to cut unnecessary calories.

It is very important, however, to realize that portion control matters too. It is still possible to overeat on low-fat foods because you're still getting calories from carbohydrate and/or protein. In other words, it wouldn't be wise to buy a box of low-fat or reduced-fat cookies and eat half the box in one sitting because they still contain calories from carbohydrate and you wouldn't be practicing moderation. Therefore, **moderation is the key** and it's important to cut back on **all** unnecessary calories, whether they come from carbohydrate, protein, or fat.

Let me emphasize this point because a critically important part of weight management is the practice of moderation critically. **If you will simply try to make healthier choices overall** (which this book will help you learn to do), **stop eating when you're not hungry between meals, and stop eating when you're full at each meal, then you will be well on your way to a healthy weight**. You may want to read the previous sentence again because you can eat "healthy" foods and still be overweight. It all comes down to MODERATION. Seriously, if you will simply stop eating when you're full at meals, which means you'll have to leave food on your plate most of the time, then you will save a significant amount of calories over time and will most certainly lose weight (assuming that you often eat past the feeling of fullness).

Earlier I mentioned that the key to weight loss is a net loss of calories; however, I don't want to only teach you how to lose weight. Instead, I want to teach you how to lose weight *and* to eat healthier, so that ultimately you will achieve both a healthier weight and a healthier body. Therefore, you must know that the **three keys to a healthy diet are:**

- ❖ **Variety**
- ❖ **Balance**
- ❖ **Moderation**

*Variety* in your diet means that you choose different foods from all of the food groups; *balance* means that you eat appropriate amounts of each food group so that one doesn't crowd out another; and *moderation* means that you don't overdo it.

## *Deceptive Labeling*

You may have noticed that products labeled "Fat Free" often have added sugar (carbohydrate) and products labeled "Sugar Free" often have added fat. This occurs because if you take one out, something else needs to be added back for flavor and/or texture. As a result, I suggest you choose "Reduced Fat," "Low-fat," or "Light" foods rather than "Fat Free" or "Sugar Free." Now, there are some fat-free items that I do recommend, such as skim milk. My point is that labeling can be deceiving. Plus, it's too tempting to eat more of something simply because it's "Fat Free" or "Sugar Free."

It's not necessary to force yourself to only buy low-fat foods; just be sure to limit your intake of high-fat foods, such as bacon, sausage, bologna, gravy, creamy sauces, regular salad dressings, and fried foods. Similarly, you don't need to focus on ridding your diet of sugar, but it would be wise to cut back on or limit your intake of sugary foods, such as regular soda and other sugary drinks, candy, snack cakes, cookies, pies, and other sweets. This is especially true if those foods are displacing healthier foods or if they're causing you to consume too many calories.

Remember that there's no need to try and completely rid your diet of an entire food group or calorie source because you need all three (carbohydrate, protein, and fat) in order to have a healthy diet. Instead, just learn where you tend to consume unnecessary calories and cut back.

## *Spending More Calories*

Okay, now let's talk more about spending some of those calories in physical activity. I'm not suggesting that you buy a room full of exercise equipment. I am suggesting, however, that you start thinking of ways to become more active. Of course, I am obligated to give you the typical "speak with your doctor before you start an exercise program" line, but I think it's safe to say that if you are generally a healthy person with no limits from your doctor on physical activity, you should be able to gradually add physical activity to your life in a safe way.

If you are wheel-chair bound due to your weight, additional activity could be as simple as lifting soup cans and doing leg lifts. Otherwise, it could mean simply walking around your house or to the mailbox, cleaning your house, gardening, taking the stairs instead of an elevator, parking farther away in parking lots, or walking around your neighborhood or the track at a nearby school or community center. Take dance lessons, play a recreational sport that you enjoy, join an aerobics class, swim, chase your child or grandchild in your backyard or at the park, walk around the shopping mall, and so on. There are many ways to incorporate physical activity into your life; anything that gets your body moving is physical activity.

Reach for a goal of half an hour of physical activity a day most days of the week, but if you aren't currently active and that seems like a lot, remember that **some is better than none.** Focus on trying to keep yourself busy and limit the time you spend watching TV or sitting at the computer.

Again, I suggest that you add activity gradually at a reasonable rate, because just like the diet, if you add too much too quickly you are more likely to suffer from burnout and eventually quit altogether. For example, if you plan to start walking, start with as little as five minutes three days a week and after the first week, add a minute each time so that in ten weeks you will have worked up to a 30-minute walk. A great way to become more active is to limit the time you spend in sedentary activities, such as watching TV, playing video games, reading, or sitting at the computer. If you have a job that requires you to sit most of the day, take a short break every hour or two and take a brisk walk around. If you have a stairway close-by, take a trip up and back down a flight or two. Remind yourself that **every bit of physical activity you do spends calories and helps move you toward your weight loss goal.**

## *Food Groups*

Okay, let's get back to nutrition. As I mentioned earlier, I want to give you some background information on what composes a healthy diet. This will help you understand where each tip fits into the scheme of things because all of the tips included in this book are based on the Dietary Guidelines for Americans and the Food Pyramid (developed by the USDA and the Department of Health and Human Services). I've included a picture of the Food Pyramid in the Resources section for your reference.

If you're interested, there's an interactive website with the Food Pyramid at mypyramid.gov. Here you can get personalized recommendations based on your sex, height, weight, and activity level. Below is an overview of each food group, but the website also contains more detailed information. If you're interested in reading more detail on the Dietary Guidelines for Americans, you can find them online at http://mypramid.gov/guidelines.

The Food Pyramid shows five basic food groups in the proportions that should comprise our diet. The five basic food groups are: **1. Grains, 2. Vegetables, 3. Fruits, 4. Milk, and 5. Meat & Beans.** A healthy diet includes a variety of foods from all of the food groups because each group provides unique nutrients. Following is a brief overview of each food group. You'll notice that I've listed the number of servings needed for each group daily and the serving sizes, but that's not because I think you should be imprisoned by numbers and measurements. Rather, it's just to give you a basic idea of how much you need to meet your nutrient needs and to give you a baseline for your current diet.

If you look at the Food Pyramid, you'll notice that **Grains** make up the largest part of it, meaning that most (or at least half) of our calories should come from those foods daily. Grains include bagels, English muffins, tortillas, oatmeal, crackers, cereal, pasta, and rice. Most women need 5–6 servings daily and most men need 6–8. A serving in the grain group is one slice of bread, half of a bagel or English muffin, four to six crackers, 1/2 cup of cooked pasta, rice, and cereal.

One thing to understand about servings is not that you should only eat one serving at a time, but rather when you eat more than one serving it simply gets counted toward your total for the day. (Note: I've only included serving sizes in this book so that you can better evaluate what foods you may need more or less of in order to meet your nutrient needs.)

**When you make choices in the grain group, it is important to concentrate on whole grains** (e.g., whole wheat breads, pastas, and cereals; brown rice; and oatmeal) rather than the processed white versions where most of the fiber and nutrients have been stripped away. Whole grains are a good source of B vitamins, iron, and magnesium and are a great source of fiber, which has many health benefits (e.g., helps lower cholesterol and reduces risk of heart disease; keeps the digestive tract swept clean and reduces constipation, the risk of diverticulosis, and the risk of colon cancer).

**Vegetables** can be divided into two groups: starchy and non-starchy. Starchy vegetables include potatoes, peas, corn, dry beans, and winter squash. Non-starchy vegetables include all others, such as broccoli, cucumber, cauliflower, peppers, carrots, spinach, green beans, tomatoes, zucchini, and many more. Contrary to popular belief (as a result of the low-carb craze), the starchy vegetables are not bad for you. In fact, they offer many nutrients and play an important role in a healthy diet. However, they are a bit higher in calories than non-starchy vegetables, so I would suggest you focus on having a combination of both daily.

For example, if you were going to have a baked potato as a side dish, I would suggest adding a tossed salad and some steamed broccoli (or any other non-starchy veggies) instead of corn and peas. This way, you'll have a combination of starchy and non-starchy veggies in your meal. A varied veggie intake will also help broaden your nutrient intake since different veggies offer different nutrients. Some of the nutrients provided by vegetables include potassium, vitamins A, C, and E, fiber, and folic acid. Plus, most vegetables are very low in fat, sodium, and calories, and have no cholesterol.

Overall, **you need 4–6 servings from the vegetable group daily.** A serving is considered 1/2 cup cooked or raw chopped, 1/2 cup (4 oz.) juice, and 1 cup raw leafy. The healthiest options in the vegetable group are those that are brightly colored because they contain higher amounts of disease-fighting antioxidants. Examples include green leafy veggies (e.g., spinach, kale, collard greens, romaine or red-leaf lettuce), carrots, broccoli, and peppers. When making a salad, choose leafy greens instead of iceberg lettuce because they have more nutrients in them. If you really like the crunch of iceberg lettuce, then at least add some spinach leaves or a leafy lettuce of some kind as a compromise. I'm a picky vegetable eater, so I try to sneak vegetables into entrees. For example, I often add finely chopped zucchini, spinach and/or yellow squash to my pasta sauce for spaghetti, baked ziti or lasagna. You can also use your food processor to finely chop veggies and add them to soups. See the Tips section for more ways to add veggies to your diet.

The **Fruit** group includes fresh fruit, canned, dried, and 100% fruit juice and you need at least 3–4 servings per day. A serving is considered 1/2 cup canned or fresh chopped, 1/2 cup (4 oz.) juice, 1 small piece of fresh fruit (e.g., a baseball-sized apple, peach, or nectarine), and 1/4 cup dried. Fruit provides potassium, vitamin C, folic acid, and fiber; is virtually free of sodium and fat; and completely free of cholesterol. I would suggest you **choose fresh fruit or fruit canned in its own juice or in light syrup** as those versions pack fewer calories than dried fruit, fruit canned in heavy syrup, and fruit juice.

If you do choose juice, however, make sure it's **100% fruit juice** and limit yourself to four to six ounces per day. When I drink juice (other than orange), I usually dilute it with water to add volume and cut the calories (or at least spread them out). For the most part, avoid fruit "drinks," "beverages," or "cocktails" as they are less nutritious and offer mostly sugar, which provides empty calories. However, I do think it's okay to choose the "Light" juice cocktails (e.g., Welch's® Light Grape Juice with added calcium) because they're lower in calories. Lastly, beware of trail mixes or other dried fruit mixes, unless you can limit yourself to a small serving (1/4 cup), because their calories add up quickly.

Fruits and veggies are packed full of powerful disease-fighters, so it's very important to add more of them to your diet in place of some of the other less nutrient-dense foods that you may be eating now. If you will start to include more fruits and veggies in your meals and snacks, you will be on your way to having a healthy blood pressure, healthy eyes and skin, a stronger immune system, and a reduced risk for many chronic health problems. They will also help you to maintain a healthy weight since they provide a feeling of fullness (from the fiber) and are low in calories.

The **Milk** group includes milk (surprise), yogurt, cheese, and cottage cheese as well as pudding (made with milk, of course), frozen yogurt, and ice cream. Remember that cheese and cottage cheese are also good sources of protein and can even replace meat in a meal occasionally. A serving is considered 1 cup milk and yogurt (8 oz.) and 1 1/2 oz. cheese (approximately 2 slices or 1/3 cup shredded). It's widely known that the milk group provides calcium and other minerals that help prevent osteoporosis, but research is beginning to show that three servings per day also helps with weight management. For weight management, you should **choose**

**low-fat or fat-free milk products**, which I discuss in the Tips section.

The **Meat & Beans** group includes meat (e.g., pork and beef), poultry, fish, dry beans and peas, eggs, nuts, and seeds. You only *need* approximately 5–6 ounces of meat or meat alternative each day in order to help meet your body's need for protein, B vitamins, iron, and zinc. Although 5–6 ounces a day doesn't seem like much, you can include more and still stay within your calorie range if you're more physically active. One egg, one tablespoon of peanut butter, 1/4 cup cooked dry beans or tofu, and 1/2 ounce of nuts or seeds are all equal to one ounce of meat, fish, or poultry (MFP). As I mentioned earlier, cheese and cottage cheese are also good sources of protein, so 1/4 cup cottage cheese or an ounce of cheese is equivalent to an ounce of MFP. Therefore, if you substitute beans or cottage cheese for meat in a meal, 3/4 cup of beans or 3/4 cup low-fat cottage cheese would provide as much protein as a 3-oz. chicken breast.

Try to limit your meat portions to the size to a deck of cards or the palm of a woman's hand. That may not sound like much because Americans generally over-consume meat. The average steak in a restaurant is at least eight ounces. Rather than considering meat the main part of your meal, consider it an accompaniment or a side and focus on having more fruits, vegetables, and whole grains instead. For weight management, you want to **choose lean meats trimmed of fat and limit your portions**. You can find examples of lean meats, fish, and poultry in the Tips section.

If you will strive to eat adequate amounts from each of the basic food groups, you'll have less room for some of the not-so-healthy foods that may be contributing to your weight.

You'll notice that the smallest/thinnest group is **Oils & Fats** (found on MyPyramid between Fruits and Milk). Although they play a role in a healthy diet, they should be consumed sparingly due to their high calorie content. The healthier choices in this group include nuts, seeds, some fish (e.g., salmon, tuna, and trout), and vegetable oils because they contain mostly unsaturated fat or "good fat." Unsaturated fats are those that do not raise cholesterol levels or contribute to heart disease and are usually liquid at room temperature.

Saturated fat, on the other hand, is the "bad fat" that does raise cholesterol and increases your risk for heart disease and stroke. Saturated fat is found mostly in solid fats, such as butter, shortening, and animal fat (e.g., the fat on the edge of a pork chop or steak or the skin on chicken).

Trans fat, which has become more popular in the media and is now included on labels, is also a type of fat that raises cholesterol levels and the risk for heart disease/stroke. Trans fat is found mainly in hard margarines (sticks) and shortenings. Products that contain hydrogenated oils as the first ingredient contain larger amounts of trans fat. As far as the margarine vs. butter debate, my suggestion is to find a soft margarine (in a tub) labeled "No Trans Fat."

## *Discretionary Calories*

In addition to the basic food groups, a healthy diet also has an allowance for discretionary calories. Discretionary calories are treats or extra calories above and beyond your basic needs (typically in the form of fat or sugar). The mypramid.gov website explains it very well in that you can think of your calorie allowance like your financial budget. You have basic costs, such as rent and food and then you have extra costs, such as movies and vacations. Your body requires a minimum number of calories from the basic food groups in order to meet its needs for nutrients; these are like the basic costs. Your extra costs or discretionary calories are treats, such as extra fat, sugar, or alcohol (e.g., regular soda, candy bars, doughnuts, cookies, cakes, pies, brownies, French fries, beer, and potato chips).

Most people have between 100–400 discretionary calories to spend daily, depending on their activity level, which means that the more active you are the more discretionary calories you are allowed. You can choose to spend your discretionary calories however you want, but remember that the better choices you make in your diet overall, the more room you have for treats. If given the option of grilled chicken or fried chicken, you could choose to spend some of your discretionary calories on the extra fat in the fried chicken, or you could choose the grilled chicken and save your discretionary calories for a few bites of dessert instead. I wouldn't suggest that you get too caught up in counting the number of discretionary calories you consume. Rather, I just want to help you understand that **treats are okay in moderation and that they can be included in a healthy diet.**

Treats are not inherently bad. The problem occurs when treats displace nutrient-rich foods (from the basic food groups) so much so that

- ❖ nutrient needs aren't met and
- ❖ calorie intake is too high.

In relationship to the financial budget mentioned above, this would be like spending too much money on movies and vacations so that there's not enough left for rent and food. Your body suffers when you don't put the right amount of nutrients into it. Most people don't even consider what nutrients their body needs when they decide what to eat. Rather, many people choose foods based only on what sounds or looks good at the time. **Learn to make healthier choices in each of the food groups in order to meet your nutrient needs without consuming too many calories. The tips in this book do exactly that; they encourage you to meet your nutrient needs as well as help you cut unnecessary calories.**

With regards to discretionary calories, it's also important to limit your intake of alcoholic beverages. Alcohol provides enough calories that it can be compared to fat in your diet. Remember that fat provides 9 cals/gram and, similarly, alcohol provides 7 cals/gram. If you drink alcohol, do so in moderation and consider it your dessert or count it as half of your evening snack. Moderate intake of alcohol is considered one drink per day for females and up to two drinks per day for males.

## *Serving Sizes*

Next, let me discuss serving sizes. I really don't believe it's necessary to measure out portions at your meals. Instead, I think you should be able to choose from a variety of food groups spaced over three meals and eat until you're full. However, if you have no idea how much you need from each food group in order to meet your nutrient needs, then it is nice to have a general guide. It's also useful to know what the recommended serving sizes are so that you can evaluate how well you're meeting your nutrient needs. For these reasons, I've provided a chart in the Sample Meal Pattern within the Resources section.

Once you know what counts as a serving, it's not hard to see how you could easily consume an adequate amount from each group. For example, 1 cup of oatmeal at breakfast, a sandwich on whole wheat bread at lunch, and 1 cup of whole wheat pasta at dinner would provide the recommended number of servings of grains (six) for the day. If nothing else, use this chart to help you determine where your diet currently stands. In order to do this, keep a food record of everything you eat and drink, including the amounts, for a few typical days. Using this chart, determine how many servings you are consuming from each group on a regular basis. Then you will have a better idea of what you need more or less of in your diet. See the Sample Food Record Evaluation within the Resources section for an example of how to evaluate your diet.

## *What is a healthy weight?*

As I've said, I think it's important for you to focus more on becoming healthier, providing your body with what it needs to function properly, and the weight loss (if needed) will occur naturally. However, if you have no idea what a healthy weight is for you, then here is a formula to help you figure it out:

- For females: 100 lbs. + 5 lbs. for every inch over 60 in height
- For males: 106 lbs. + 6 lbs. for every inch over 60 in height

You can add or subtract 10% based on your frame size. In other words, if you are a large frame, you can add 10% to your final number and if you're a small frame you can subtract 10%. Keep in mind that this is a very rough estimate for ideal body weight. The number you get may seem unrealistic for you, and that's fine. I don't want you to be focused on the number on the scale. Believe me, if you adopt the eating habits in this book, you will reach and maintain a healthy weight. Although it will probably come off at a slow pace (0.5–2 pounds per week), it will come off and stay off as long as you stick with it.

Another way to evaluate your weight is to look at your BMI, or Body Mass Index. BMI is simply a comparison of your weight for height. In general, as BMI increases, so does the risk for health complications. Keep in mind that the BMI is meant to compare the average body type. One of the BMI's downfalls is that it does not take into consideration your body composition, which means that if you happen to be quite muscular, then your BMI may seem falsely high. In other words, the BMI assumes that any extra weight you have is fat, not muscle.

The goal is to have a BMI less than 25 in order to decrease your risk for diseases associated with being overweight. A BMI between 18.5 and 24.9 corresponds to a healthy weight. As your weight rises above that level so does your risk for diseases, including high blood pressure, diabetes, heart disease, stroke, and some cancers. You can find a BMI calculator on both the Center for Disease Control's website at cdc.gov or the National Institutes of Health's website at nih.gov.

As I mentioned earlier, if you want to have a weight loss goal, I suggest that you start with a 10% weight loss and limit weigh-ins to once per week at most. Weighing yourself too often causes you to concentrate too much on the number on the scale and leads to discouragement if you don't lose as quickly as you would like. If you get discouraged easily by a slow, gradual loss, then you may want to spread out weigh-ins to once every two to three weeks. One week you might do better than another, so if you limit weigh-ins then you'll have fewer opportunities for discouragement.

When you do weigh yourself, keep it consistent by weighing at the same time of day on the same scale with the same amount of clothes on (or no clothes at all). I suggest that you weigh in the morning, before your shower, and after you use the restroom (every little bit counts). More than the number on the scale, focus on the difference you feel in your clothes and, more importantly, the difference you feel both physically and mentally. As you start to reach a healthier weight, pay attention to little things, like how you don't get winded as easily when climbing the stairs, how your hips, knees, and ankles don't hurt as much as they used to, how your blood pressure has gone down, how much more energy you have, and so on.

# *Tips*

Now that I've discussed the basics of a healthy diet, the following tips should make more sense. After you've read through them, go back and pick out one or two that you can begin to work on for the next couple of weeks (or until you've mastered them). I suggest that you choose to adopt only a couple of tips at a time because making too many changes at once can be overwhelming and lead to frustration. You may be the type of person who is "all or nothing" and want to make several changes at once, but fight that temptation.

Remember, this is a marathon, not a sprint, so pace yourself and make gradual changes. Trust me—gradual changes are much more likely to lead to your success, so once you've mastered the first couple of tips, then move on to the next one, and so on. Before you know it, you will have mastered all or most of the tips and you will be following a healthy diet at a healthier weight. I recommend you **go back and read these paragraphs again, because I feel their message is vitally important. I know you want to lose weight as quickly as possible, but remember how long it took you to put it on. It didn't**

**happen in two weeks, so realize that it's going to take some time to take it off.**

As you begin this journey, please realize that you are going to "mess up" at times because you are not perfect; everyone makes mistakes. Even after years of practice, I eat more than I should now and then. It is very important that you do not let these blunders keep you down. Try not to let them happen very often, but when they do, realize your mistake and try harder at your next meal; whatever you do, don't give up! Really, there's no need to give up because this is not a diet, this is your new way of eating for life. Keep your head up and your eyes on your goal. Remember that winners aren't those who never make mistakes but those who learn from them and keep going in spite of them (okay, so that may have been a bit cliché, but it's true!).

As you read further into the tips, you may feel that some of them seem like such small, insignificant changes, and you may be inclined to think that it won't make enough of a difference, but remember that **a lot of small changes make a big change when they're put together.** If you want to see results, trust me and commit to follow these tips as closely as possible. I hope you're excited about the changes you are about to make in your diet. If you stick with them, you'll be on your way to a healthy weight and a healthier life. Let's begin, shall we?

# (1)

**Eat three regular meals every day.** Whatever you do, DO NOT SKIP MEALS because it leads to overeating later. Try to space your meals approximately four to six hours apart. When you allow too much time between meals you're more likely to overeat. On the other hand, if you eat too often throughout the day, you're less likely to be hungry enough to eat a well-rounded meal. Get yourself on a regular schedule.

This is the first tip because it's an extremely important one; make it your first priority. Nine times out of ten the patients I've seen for weight loss didn't eat on a regular schedule, so that's the first thing we worked on. One of the biggest mistakes you can make when trying to cut calories is to skip a meal. It's important to keep your metabolism "fired up;" eating on a regular schedule is like adding wood to a fire. Remember that your body was designed to survive if faced with a famine, so when you go long periods without food, your metabolism lowers in order to conserve energy. You need to start your day with breakfast and then eat about every four to six hours.

Having three meals on a regular schedule and eating until you're full at each meal will also help reduce your cravings for snacks. If you're someone who tends to eat continually from dinner until bedtime, it's most likely because you aren't eating enough throughout the day and your body is trying to make up for lost calories.

I've included a week's worth of sample menus from my own diet in the Resources section so that you will have a general idea of what an appropriate diet looks like in regards to types, proportion, and timing of food. Keep in mind that the amount of food you need is based on your individual calorie needs, so follow your body's lead rather than feeling as if you should eat the exact amounts I've listed.

## (2)

**Plan ahead.** If you have a plan, it's much easier to make the right choices. Try not to wait until you're hungry to decide what to eat. Once you've gotten to the point of hunger, you are much more likely to make irrational decisions and eat whatever looks good. Believe me, I've done this myself. Have you ever stood in front of the pantry, nibbling on this and that while you try to decide what to make? Instead, sit down and plan balanced meals a day or even a week in advance.

I plan out my dinners for the week and then make my grocery list based on them. Not only does this improve the chances of having healthier meals, it also saves money at the grocery store. I don't actually plan out each breakfast and lunch in detail, but do make sure I have healthy options for each. See the Resources section for a Sample Grocery List based on a week's plan for meals.

Planning ahead doesn't mean that you have to prepare extravagant meals. Take advantage of ready-prepared items at the grocery store, like bagged salads, bagged veggie mixes, pre-chopped fresh fruit, and so on. If you don't feel like cooking when you get home from work, try using a slow cooker. The fast food restaurant on the way home won't be nearly as tempting when you know you have a hot, well- balanced meal waiting on you.

    Decide what you're going to have at your next meal before you even get hungry and have it ready to eat by the time you get hungry. For example, if you tend to eat lunch at noon, start thinking about what you're going to have around 11:00am or so and then have it ready by noon so that you aren't scrambling for something to eat at the last minute. If you work outside the home, plan some healthy lunch foods you can take to work with you instead of eating out most of the time. Taking your lunch to work can save a significant amount of calories. If you travel for work, try packing a cooler to take with you in order to reduce the amount you eat out. See the Sample Menus within the Resources section for ideas.

## (3)

**Stop eating when you're full.** I truly believe that this is one of the most important tips for weight loss, which is why it made the top three. This sounds intuitive, but for most people it's a very difficult thing to do. You've learned to push past that feeling of fullness because the food tastes good, it's a habit, or you don't want the food to go to waste. As a child you were probably made to clean your plate whether you were full or not. Unfortunately, this practice teaches children to ignore the satiety signal from their brain that says they're full.

Restaurants tend to give large portions and most people feel the need to finish all of it. It's time to start listening to your body—**when your stomach feels full, push your plate away.** Before you get a second helping, ask yourself, "Am I still hungry or do I just want to eat more?" If you're actually starting to feel full, push that plate away; remind yourself that you can have a snack later in the evening. Don't let yourself eat to the point that your stomach feels uncomfortable, like you need to unbutton your pants or loosen your belt. Just think of how many calories you will save if you start pushing your plate away when you're full. It may seem like those few extra bites are insignificant, but extra bites at every meal will add up over time. Before you know it, you will have lost pounds just from that one change.

If you are at a restaurant, take part of the meal home so it's not wasted if that's an issue for you, or split a meal with someone (it's cheaper that way anyway). You can also try ordering from the kid's menu in order to start with a smaller portion. Interestingly, the kids' portions in restaurants these days are similar to the adult portions served 50 years ago. If you are compelled to finish your plate, then start with smaller portions than usual or use a smaller plate.

Here's an interesting point: the better you are at stopping when you're full, the more lenient you can be in your food choices. If you tend to overeat often, it's very important that you choose lower calorie foods in order to still lose weight; however, as you gain more self control and get good at pushing your plate away even when there are just a few bites left, you will have the freedom to choose higher calorie foods more often. For example, one of my favorite treat foods is French fries. When at a restaurant, I sometimes order them as a side to my meal or to share with my family because I am confident in my ability to stop when I'm full. However, if I didn't trust myself to be satisfied with only a handful of them, then I just wouldn't order them.

Not only do you want to stop eating before you're uncomfortably full, you also don't want to stop eating *before* you're full because then you'll be more tempted to snack between meals. You don't want to leave the table uncomfortably full and you also don't want to leave the table still hungry. It will take some practice to learn what level of fullness is enough to keep you satisfied until your next meal without overdoing it. Since you'll be having three meals per day, you'll have plenty of opportunities to practice. Once you've mastered this tip, you will feel such gratification because you will be in control of your appetite rather than your appetite in control of you.

# (4)

**Make time for breakfast.** You've heard this one for a long time and it's true—breakfast is very important to a healthy diet. It *break*s the *fast* you've had overnight and gets your metabolism "fired up." Also, studies have shown that providing your brain with fuel from breakfast allows you to think and perform better at school or work. Furthermore, eating a healthy breakfast (and lunch) helps prevent overeating later in the day. One of the most common problems I have encountered with patients seeking weight loss is that they skip breakfast and/or lunch, eat a very large dinner and then snack all evening until bedtime, as their body attempts to make up for the lost calories during the day.

Healthy breakfast options include ready-to-eat cereals with at least five grams of fiber per serving (e.g., Shredded Wheat, Mini-Wheats®, Raisin Bran, bran flakes, Fiber One®, All-Bran®, and Kashi®), oatmeal, whole grain bagels, English muffins, toast (with at least two grams of fiber per serving) with low-sugar jelly or light cream cheese, whole grain waffles or pancakes, fresh fruit, and skim milk.

A high-fiber breakfast helps you stay full until lunch without cravings for snacks. I've had the most success with cereals that have at least five grams of fiber per serving. If you don't like any of the high-fiber cereals, then try mixing one of them with your favorite. This way, you'll get to taste your favorite cereal and get extra fiber at the same time. Sometimes I mix about 1/2 cup of Fiber One® with Honey Clusters with about 2/3 cup of Cinnamon Toast Crunch®. It's all about moderation and compromise. For more breakfast ideas, see the Sample Menus within the Resources section.

If you don't feel that you have time to eat breakfast at home before work, then try to put a quick breakfast together before you go to bed. Breakfast doesn't need to be a four course meal. You could put some light cream cheese between two bagel halves and put it in a baggie, grab some orange juice or skim milk and eat on the go. Or, grab a container of yogurt and put some granola or Fiber One® on top as you head out the door. This isn't ideal and I would rather you make time to eat breakfast, but it's definitely better than not eating at all. You also don't have to eat traditional breakfast food. Try a ham and cheese sandwich on whole wheat bread with a banana and some milk or orange juice. Another quick and easy breakfast is Jimmy Dean's D-Lights® breakfast sandwiches found in the frozen foods section of the grocery store.

## (5)

**Get more fiber.** Fiber has so many great benefits and is absolutely essential to a healthy diet. Fiber is the part of fruits, vegetables, and grains that doesn't get digested; it actually travels through your entire digestive system and out. Since we don't have the enzymes to break down fiber, we can't absorb it, which means we don't get calories from it. It actually slows down the early digestive process in the stomach, which helps to keep you full longer. Fiber also slows the rate at which your blood sugar rises after a meal.

Fiber has been shown to lower cholesterol levels, as well as reduce the risk for heart disease and colon cancer. Since it adds bulk to your stool, it reduces the risk of diverticulosis (pouches in the colon), constipation, and hemorrhoids. Lastly, fiber increases the production of "good bacteria" in the colon, which helps the immune system.

Breakfast is a great time to fit in a good amount of fiber, but try to squeeze more fiber in throughout the rest of the day too by eating fruits and vegetables (with the skin when possible) as well as whole grains. Look on the label for fiber content (under Total Carbohydrate); try to find grains (e.g., breads, tortillas, rice, pasta, bagels, English muffins, waffles, and buns) that have at least two grams of fiber per serving. Try to find a breakfast cereal that has at least five grams of fiber per serving. Beans are also a great source of fiber, so add them to meals when you can. Whenever I make a Mexican dish, I always add a can of beans to the meat, whether it's ground beef or chicken. You can also add beans to many of your soups and casseroles.

Adults need 20–35 grams of fiber per day. Your kiddos need about five grams plus one gram for each year of age. Be sure to increase your fiber intake gradually and drink more fluids to help decrease the potential side effects.

## (6)

**Limit sugary drinks.** These include regular soda, fruity drinks, like Kool-Aid®, Hi-C®, lemonade, sweet tea, and sweetened coffee drinks. Sugary drinks only provide empty calories, meaning that you get little or no nutrient value from them. In addition, liquid calories aren't nearly as satisfying as food, so your stomach and brain don't recognize that you've gotten a significant number of calories. If you cut the calories in your drinks, you'll have more room for food in your total calorie allowance.

Drinks are such a quick, easy way to cut unnecessary calories, which is why it's always one of my first suggestions for anyone who wants to lose weight. Choose low-calorie or sugar-free beverages, such as water, diet soda in moderation, Crystal Light® or equivalent, diet lemonade, unsweetened or artificially sweetened tea or coffee, and so on. If you do choose fruit juice or sweetened tea, dilute them with water in order to cut the calories.

Other than 2–3 cups of low-fat milk and up to 6 ounces of 100% fruit juice per day, choose beverages with around 15 calories or less per serving; check the label to make sure. Also, if you normally sweeten beverages with sugar, you could switch to an artificial sweetener, such as Splenda® or Equal®. Start paying attention to how many liquid calories you're consuming; you may be surprised because they add up quickly. Here's a fun fact: if you currently drink three to four cans of regular soda per day and switch to a low-calorie beverage, you will lose approximately one pound per week just from that one change!

# (7)

**Have three servings of calcium-rich foods daily.** We've known for a long time that calcium is important for the prevention of osteoporosis. In addition, recent studies have shown that those who consume adequate calcium in foods and beverages (as opposed to supplements) are better able to maintain a healthy weight. In order to cut calories, choose low-fat dairy products, such as skim or 1% milk, low-fat yogurt, cheeses made from 2% milk (when possible), calcium-fortified orange juice and soy milk, and firm tofu. A serving is considered one cup of milk or orange juice (8 oz.), a 6–8 oz. container of yogurt, and 1.5 ounces of cheese (2 slices or 1/3 cup shredded). I usually have skim milk or calcium-fortified orange juice with breakfast, low-fat yogurt or a slice of cheese with lunch, and a cup of skim milk with my evening snack (usually in cereal).

For those who are lactose intolerant or have a milk allergy, the calcium-fortified juices are a good option. Studies have shown that our bones absorb the calcium from those just as well as from dairy products.

## (8)

**Slow down.** Take time to enjoy your meal. The more you are able to savor the food, the more enjoyable it will be, and the more satisfied you will feel. Rather than eating on the go, while watching TV, or while running around the house, take the time to sit and eat your meal or snack. When you aren't distracted during a meal, your brain registers that you've gotten calories and you won't feel as if you need to continue grazing throughout the day. There have been times when I've made lunch for my kiddos and then ate my lunch while cleaning up the kitchen or putting dishes away. Those lunches aren't nearly as satisfying and I'm more tempted to snack soon afterwards.

Have a conversation with someone during your meal, put your fork down occasionally, take drinks, and chew more. If you eat quickly, you will end up consuming more food/calories than you need before you realize you're full. You may have heard before that it takes your brain approximately 20 minutes to realize you're full, so the longer you take to eat the less you will need to eat in order to feel full. Therefore, try to make your meal last longer.

## (9)

**Choose healthier snacks.** A couple of healthy snacks each day can actually be a good thing. If you are truly hungry between meals, a small healthy snack can help prevent overeating at your next meal. If you go into a meal feeling extra hungry, you're more likely to overeat. It's especially important to include a small snack if you have a long period of time between meals (although it would be best to try and plan for meals to be spaced approximately 4–6 hours apart).

Some diets encourage you to stop eating after a certain time in the evening (e.g., 6:00 or 7:00pm). Research has shown, however, that your weight is more related to your total calorie intake for the day. In other words, allowing yourself to have a reasonable evening snack is not, in itself, going to cause weight gain. In my house, we almost always have an evening snack between dinner and bedtime. I think it helps you to not overeat at dinner because you know that you have that evening snack to look forward to. Make sure you only have one snack, however. I know it's common for people to eat several snacks in the evening out of enjoyment or boredom. If you will eat three meals throughout the day on a regular schedule, however, it should help reduce your "need" to snack as much in the evening. Remember that skipping meals earlier in the day causes you to overeat later as your body (and mind) attempt to make up for lost calories.

Make sure you choose the right snack foods. Buy less of the high-fat, high-sugar snacks that tempt you daily (e.g., potato chips, snack cakes, candy bars, doughnuts). That's not to say that you should never eat these foods, but they should only be eaten in moderation. If you have a hard time controlling your intake of them, then try not to buy them very often. If they aren't staring you in the face every day, it will be much easier to avoid them. One healthier chip option would be to try the baked or lower-fat version (e.g., Baked Doritos®, Baked Cheetos®, Baked Lay's®), but remember to stick to one portion at a time. Don't be tempted to eat more of a food just because it's labeled as "low-fat" or "sugar-free" because that defeats the purpose of choosing those foods to save calories. Also, be sure to check the label to compare the calorie content of the regular version versus the baked or low-fat version. If the low-fat or reduced-fat version isn't that much different, then just choose the regular one.

Another way to save calories when snacking is to look at the Nutrition Label and take out the portion listed under "serving size." After you take that amount out of the container, put it back in the cabinet/pantry. Try not to sit down with the entire box or bag because you'll be less aware of how much you're eating and you'll probably eat a much larger portion.

Other healthy snack options include low-fat yogurt, fresh fruit, low-fat ice cream or frozen yogurt, low-fat cottage cheese, tortilla chips with salsa, animal crackers, a palmful of nuts (especially almonds and walnuts), vanilla wafers, ginger snaps, graham crackers, pretzels, an apple with a thin layer of peanut butter, string cheese, low-fat popcorn, a low-fat granola bar, a serving of crackers with a slice of cheese, 1/2 cup of pudding, whole wheat pita bread with hummus or other bean dip, raw vegetables with a low-fat dip, dry cereal, whole wheat toast with low-sugar jelly, a homemade fruit smoothie with yogurt and frozen berries, cereal with skim milk (one of my favorites), or half a sandwich with lean meat or peanut butter.

You may also need to work on a more regular sleep schedule, because if you tend to stay up very late at night, then you may be more tempted to eat when you aren't actually hungry, especially if you're watching TV or sitting at the computer.

If you wake up in the middle of the night, try to avoid eating. If you are actually hungry, try drinking a low-calorie beverage (see Tip #6 for ideas) or a cup of skim milk; or eat a lower calorie food, such as sugar-free JELL-O®, a slice of toast, a few crackers, or a piece of fruit.

# (10)

**Allow treats in moderation.** Another common dieting mistake is to avoid all treats. Of course, these foods (e.g., candy bars, cookies, brownies, cake, pie, French fries, onion rings, potato chips, etc.) aren't necessary for a healthy diet and they don't provide many nutrients, but they sure are tasty. These foods are not harmful if consumed in moderation. As soon as you tell yourself that you can't have something, it's all you're going to think about. Once you've gone without it for a while, you'll likely get discouraged, give up, and overindulge on it. If you know that these foods are not off-limits, they won't be nearly as big of a deal. If you were to look in my pantry right now, you would likely find some peanut M&M's®, Raisinettes®, or some mini candy bars, and some type of cookie.

Here's the trick though—keep portions small. I like M&M's® and Raisinettes® because I can grab a few to quench that chocolate craving instead of opening a candy bar or other packaged dessert and feeling compelled to eat the entire thing. If you're like me, you like to end lunch and dinner with something sweet. That's when I allow myself to have a few bites of chocolate or a couple of small cookies. An important key to eating treats in moderation is to avoid them when you're hungry. Instead, have them at the end of a meal so that you'll be satisfied with a smaller amount. If you wait until you're hungry, you might be tempted to eat the entire roll of Thin Mints®, whereas if you save it for the end of your meal, you'll be satisfied with two or three.

Another treat for me is a Blizzard® from Dairy Queen®, which I probably have once every few months or so (I'm not a big ice cream fan). I always get a small, eat half of it, and put the other half in the freezer for the next day. It's just a way to allow yourself to have a treat without overindulging. If you're used to getting a large and eating the entire amount in one sitting, then I'm not suggesting you should start getting a small and only eat half of it right away because you'll feel completely deprived and like you're on a diet. Instead, start with a medium, then move to a small, so that it's more of a gradual change and easier to maintain. Working on your self-control in small steps is more likely to lead to long-term success. If it makes it any easier for you to make the change, a small cookie dough Blizzard® has 720 calories and a medium has a whopping 1030 calories.

True self-control comes not when you make yourself completely avoid treats, but when you can be around these foods and limit yourself to a moderate amount. Again, don't sabotage your chances at moderation by eating these foods when you're really hungry because you'll eat more of them. Have them at the end of a meal so that you're satisfied with just enough to quench your craving.

When I use the term "treats" I don't just mean sweets. It's also important to allow yourself to have other sorts of treats occasionally too. Learn to make healthier choices most of the time, but it's okay to have barbecued ribs or a cheeseburger and fries for dinner now and then; simply plan for these treats by limiting calories earlier in the day. Something else you can do to help balance out the calories is to add more physical activity to your day. **Do not, however, skip a meal in an attempt to save calories.** Instead, choose lower calorie foods for the other meals (e.g., have a salad with low-fat dressing and fruit for lunch).

Also when having treats (as always), be sure to stop eating when you're full. You definitely don't want to overeat on treats because it will result in the consumption of even more unnecessary calories. If you feel like you have overeaten, then simply make it a point to either watch calories a bit closer at the next meal or the next day or do more physical activity to help spend the extra calories.

# (11)

**Eat more vegetables.** If you don't eat any vegetables (French fries and potato chips don't count), then start with one serving a day. If you eat one serving a day, then start having two, and so on until you have at least four servings or more every day. If you're picky when it comes to vegetables (like me), then try to branch out and experiment with new ones on a regular basis. Set a goal to try a new vegetable once a week; if you have kiddos, let them pick a new vegetable to try as well in order to encourage them to eat it with you. Also, if you don't like a vegetable cooked one way, try cooking it another way. Don't let your veggies get too mushy when you cook them; they aren't very appetizing and it destroys some of their nutrient content. Don't be afraid to dip your veggies in a light dip or dressing; it's better to get the many benefits of the veggies with a few extra calories than to avoid them altogether.

Try to have a serving of vegetables at lunch and then at least three at dinner. If you don't get one in at lunch, then have four at dinner. That doesn't mean you have to eat four different vegetables, just that you get four *servings* of vegetables. A serving is considered 1/2 cup cooked or chopped and 1 cup raw leafy, so if you have a medium-sized baked potato, that would count as two servings and 1 cup of cooked broccoli/cauliflower/carrot mix would also count as two servings. At a meal, try to only have one starchy vegetable (e.g., peas, corn, or potatoes) and then add another non-starchy vegetable (e.g., green beans, broccoli, carrots, cauliflower, tossed salad, Brussels sprouts, tomato, sliced cucumber, zucchini, peppers, greens, cabbage, asparagus). If you clean your plate and you're still hungry, go back for more vegetables since they're lower in calories than the other parts of the meal.

One way to make it easy to get an extra serving in is to put out some raw veggies with a low-fat dip while you're cooking dinner (this is especially good for holding your kiddos over). Plus, it helps take up some room in your stomach so you don't start your meal feeling so hungry, which means you're less likely to overeat. Another idea is to buy the bags of frozen vegetables that can either be steamed in the microwave or tossed into a pan on the stovetop. You could also buy the ready-to-use bags of salad. One of my favorite quick-and-easy products are the bags of fresh veggies (broccoli, cauliflower, and carrots) in the produce section that can be put in the microwave for just a few minutes.

Try not to add much fat to your veggies (e.g., butter, margarine, bacon grease). Instead, use a "butter" spray or cook them in chicken or vegetable broth to add a lot of flavor with very few calories. If you like to add bacon fat when cooking your veggies, use a slice of turkey bacon or ham instead. Or, you could even add a slice of regular bacon and the dish would still contain far fewer calories than adding a tablespoon or two of bacon grease. Also, if you have a tossed salad, place only a small amount of light or low-fat dressing on it or dip your fork in the dressing on the side.

# (12)

**Eat more fruit.** As vegetables go, so go fruits. If you don't eat any fruit, then start with one serving a day until you have at least three to four servings every day. Choose fresh (with the skin for fiber) or canned in water, its own juice, or light syrup. Limit fruit juice to 4-6 oz. a day and choose 100% fruit juices rather than fruit drinks, cocktails, or fruit ades (e.g., Capri Sun®, Kool-Aid®, Hi-C®, Sunny D®, Hawaiian Punch®). Typically, darker juices, such as grape and cranberry are higher in calories (unless you find a light version). Except for orange juice, I dilute all juices with water to cut the calories (2/3 juice, 1/3 water).

One easy way to eat more fruit is to make a fruit salad so it's easy to grab as a snack or a side for a meal. Or, even easier, take advantage of the ready-to-eat chopped fruit in the produce section; those make it an absolute cinch to eat more fruit. An easy way to ensure adequate fruit intake is to make it a habit to eat a serving with each meal. For example, add blueberries to your cereal, slice an apple with lunch, and have some fresh strawberries with dinner. If you focus on getting adequate amounts of fruits and vegetables, they should start to replace other less healthy options you may be eating now, which will lower your calorie intake.

## (13)

**Limit your fat intake.** In the introduction I explained that fat is the richest source of calories in our diet, so try to limit your fat intake in order to control calories. Notice I didn't recommend a "fat-free" diet because our bodies need some fat to function properly. The general recommendation is to limit fat to 30% of your calories. That's anywhere from 50–80 grams of fat per day (for 1500–2500 calorie diets) if you want to count fat grams. I don't think it's necessary to have to always count grams of fat or calories, but it's a great starting point in order to learn where extra calories may be lurking in your diet.

Once you start paying attention to how many fat grams you're consuming, you'll get a better idea as to what foods to choose less often. To get an idea of how much fat you're currently eating, start looking at the labels of the foods you choose most often and add up the fat grams. Note that the fat grams listed are for one serving, so if you eat two servings, then you need to double the grams of fat.

When you eat out, ask for a Nutrition Guide at your favorite restaurants. Many restaurants have a website that contains their nutrition information, including calories and fat grams. I often look up a restaurant's menu with nutrition information before going out to eat so I can pick an item with less calories and fat. Also, most menus indicate lower fat items with some sort of symbol; if you're not sure how to find them, just ask your server.

In general, try to choose baked or grilled items instead of fried (grilled chicken instead of fried chicken), lean meats (skinless chicken breast or sirloin instead of prime rib), low-fat dairy products (skim or 1% milk instead of 2% or whole), steamed vegetables, vegetable soup, salad with light dressing, or fruit instead of French fries or other fried items. Also limit the amount of fat you add to your foods with butter, margarine, sour cream, cream cheese, gravy, Alfredo sauce, cheese sauce, and other creamy sauces. Many of the remaining tips pertain to lowering the fat in your diet since it is such a great way to save calories.

# (14)

**Choose foods that are "light," "low-fat," or "reduced-fat."** Examples include the following: light bread (make sure it still has at least two grams of fiber per slice), light or low-fat salad dressing, light sour cream, light mayo or Miracle Whip®, light syrup, low-sugar jelly (all jelly is fat-free, but low-sugar jelly contains fewer calories from sugar), light cream cheese, reduced-fat cheese, low-fat yogurt, low-fat cottage cheese, low-fat frozen yogurt, and low-fat ice cream. In general, I don't recommend choosing "fat-free" items because they don't usually taste as good or cook as well, and they often have added sugar, which adds calories back in.

## (15)

**Use low-fat cooking methods.** Some ways to cook with less fat include the following: bake, broil, grill, steam, boil, roast, braise or stew, use the slow-cooker or pressure cooker. For the most part, avoid frying, especially deep-fat frying. If you need to cook with fat, just use a small amount of vegetable oil. The healthiest oils include canola, olive, and peanut. They aren't any lower in calories than butter or shortening, but they contain monounsaturated fat, which is heart healthy. If possible, try to get away with using a non-stick spray instead.

## (16)

**Trim fat and skin from meat and poultry.** Before you cook meat or poultry, pull or cut off all of the visible fat from the outside or edge. If you didn't prepare the meat, then just be sure to take the skin off or cut the fat away before you eat it. If you boil or roast meat or poultry and save the broth or drippings, put them in the refrigerator long enough for the fat to rise to the top and skim it off.

## (17)

**Limit high-fat meats.** Examples include bacon, sausage, spareribs, prime rib, organ meats (e.g., liver, brains, kidney), hamburger, hot dogs, bologna, salami, and pepperoni. When grocery shopping for meat, choose cuts that have very little or no white marbling throughout the meat. The more white marbling in a cut of meat, the more fat, and calories it contains.

# (18)

**Choose lean meat, fish, and poultry.** Examples include round, sirloin, and flank steak, tenderloin, lean and extra-lean ground beef or turkey (92–96% lean), skinless chicken and turkey breast, pork loin and center loin chops, tuna canned in water, salmon, ham, Canadian bacon, cod, flounder, haddock, lobster, and crab.. If you have a craving for a hot dog or smoked sausage, choose Healthy Choice® brand. You can also find turkey pepperoni, 50% less fat ground sausage, and turkey bacon. To give you an idea of the difference in calories and fat, a regular hot dog has approximately 180 calories and 16 grams of fat whereas a Healthy Choice® hot dog has 70 calories and 2.5 grams of fat. Many meats have labels on the back now, so compare labels when grocery shopping and choose the cut with fewer calories and less fat per serving.

# (19)

**Eat more legumes.** Legumes include beans, peas, and lentils. They're low in fat, cholesterol-free, high in fiber, and inexpensive. Beans are a good source of protein, which means you can substitute them for meat. Have beans in place of meat on a regular basis, such as weekly or biweekly.

This is easy to do in Mexican dishes, casseroles, and soups. For example, if you are planning to make chicken quesadillas, leave out the chicken and replace it with black beans or pinto beans instead. Don't forget to season the beans just as you would have seasoned the chicken (i.e., with taco seasoning). Also, if you have a soup recipe that calls for ground beef, simply leave out the beef and replace it with a variety of beans (e.g., Great Northern®, pinto, navy, or kidney). Even if you don't want to replace the meat in a meal, go ahead and add some beans for their health benefits.

# (20)

### Have a meatless dinner at least once a week.

This reduces calories, saturated fat, and cholesterol. As a substitute for meat, choose low-fat cottage cheese, 2% milk cheese (if available), tofu, or legumes. For example, you could have cheese tortellini, cheese ravioli, or whole wheat pasta with tomato sauce along with a tossed salad and light garlic bread (New York® Lite Garlic Toast is my favorite). If you can't find light garlic bread, simply scrape some of the garlic butter off the bread before baking.

Other meatless meal ideas include vegetable, potato, split pea or bean soup with cornbread and a side of fresh sliced cucumbers and tomatoes, or a baked potato with a side of mixed vegetables and low-fat cottage cheese. My husband likes to put cottage cheese on top of his potato, which saves calories from butter or sour cream. I, on the other hand, use a small amount of trans fat-free margarine for the middle of the potato and then barbecue or steak sauce for the outer part.

# (21)

**Eat, drink, and cook with low-fat dairy products.** Examples include skim or 1% milk; light, low-fat, or fat-free yogurt; 2% milk cheeses; and low-fat cottage cheese. If you normally use evaporated milk (e.g., Milnot®), half and half or heavy cream in a recipe, try fat-free evaporated milk instead. If you don't like the taste of skim milk, try "Skim Deluxe." It's a thicker version that tastes more like 2%. Drinking one cup (8 oz.) of 2% milk is like adding a teaspoon of butter to a cup of skim milk. If you currently drink three cups of 2% milk per day and switch to skim, you could lose approximately nine pounds in a year from that one small change. *Note: Children need whole milk (vitamin D) until the age of two for adequate fat intake.*

# (22)

**Use low-fat or light condiments.** Examples include light sour cream, light cream cheese, light mayonnaise or Miracle Whip®, and reduced-fat, light, or low-fat salad dressings. If you like tartar sauce, make your own using light mayo. Non-creamy condiments, like ketchup, mustard, barbecue sauce, salsa, and steak sauce are all low-fat choices as well.

# (23)

**Top baked potatoes with low-fat or fat-free toppings.** Examples include barbecue sauce, steak sauce, salsa, light Ranch dressing, non-fat yogurt (a great substitute for sour cream), light sour cream, low-fat cottage cheese, broccoli and 2% milk shredded cheddar cheese, pump-spray "butter", Butter Buds®, or Molly McButter®. If you really like butter on your baked potato, use a trans fat-free margarine in moderation (i.e., 1–2 teaspoons). Make sure to eat the skin of your potato too, as it contains nutrients and fiber.

# (24)

**Top pasta with tomato-based sauces.** Traditional red pasta sauces are much lower in fat and calories than white creamy sauces, such as Alfredo. I like to put diced, Italian-seasoned tomatoes in my food processor and add them to sautéed onion and garlic for a quick, healthy pasta sauce. I sometimes toss mushrooms, green pepper, zucchini and yellow squash into the food processor along with the tomatoes to add more nutrients to the sauce. The food processor allows you to add veggies to your diet that you may not even like since it chops them so finely. You can barely tell they're in the sauce, but your body gets the benefits of their nutrients.

If you prefer to buy ready-made pasta sauce, you can find lower calorie varieties in the grocery store, like

Ragu® Light and Healthy Choice® brand. If you really like white creamy sauce, find a recipe and make your own light version using half the amount of butter called for and substitute fat-free evaporated milk for the heavy cream.

# (25)

**Choose clear soups over creamy ones.** Soups such as minestrone, vegetable, bean, and chicken noodle are generally lower in calories than their creamy counterparts, such as cream of broccoli, cream of mushroom, or cream of potato. Again, you could make your own "creamy" soups using fat-free evaporated or skim milk. When I make potato soup, I thicken it with a roux made from trans fat-free margarine and flour. I also add some 2% milk shredded cheddar cheese, again for thickening and flavor, and then add skim milk for the bulk of the soup. If you want a more buttery flavor, you can add some artificial butter flavor (found in the spice isle at the grocery store).

# (26)

**Use more egg whites than yolks.** Not only do the yolks contain the cholesterol, they also contain about three times as many calories as the whites. You don't need to completely eliminate yolks from your diet, but if you eat four or more yolks per week, cut at least half of them. When I make tuna salad, I use all of the egg whites and only half the yolks. For scrambled eggs or an omelet use one whole egg plus two egg whites. You can buy egg substitutes (e.g., Egg Beaters®), but I prefer to just toss the unused yolks down the drain (it's cheaper that way). By the way, egg substitutes are basically just egg whites with color added.

In most recipes you can substitute two whites for one whole egg. Think of the egg in two parts, the yolk and the white—if you take the yolk out, it takes two whites to equal one whole egg. Some recipes won't turn out well if you substitute all the yolks for whites, because yolks provide color, flavor, and texture. Therefore, if a recipe calls for two eggs or more, substitute whites for only half of the yolks. For example, if a recipe calls for four eggs, you could use two whole eggs and four egg whites.

# (27)

## Compare calories on the Nutrition Label.

Sometimes a lower fat version (especially a fat-free version) has just as many calories as the regular version. As you are probably aware, fat adds a nice flavor and texture to many foods, so when the fat is taken out of a product, another ingredient is usually added in order to make the product acceptable. The substitute ingredient is generally sugar, which adds calories back in. For example, regular peanut butter has approximately 190 calories per serving and reduced-fat peanut butter has the exact same number of calories. That means there is no advantage in buying the reduced-fat version as far as weight management is concerned. Similarly, when sugar is taken out of a product fat is often added back in, which is why "Sugar-Free" products are often high in fat. Remember that weight management is all about calories, so despite claims of sugar-free or fat-free on the front of the package, don't forget to turn it around and compare the number of calories per serving.

# (28)

**Use less butter and/or margarine.** Butter and regular margarine have around 35 calories per teaspoon and 105 calories per tablespoon. Fun fact: if you were to cut out just one teaspoon of butter a day, you would lose four pounds of fat in a year from that one tiny change! If you always add butter to your bread, dinner rolls, muffins, corn bread, toast, corn, green beans, and carrots, try a pump-spray "butter" instead. You could also try a whipped or light, trans fat-free margarine in order to save some calories, or even one of those spreads that have actually been shown to lower cholesterol levels (Benecol® and Smart Balance®).

You can almost always cut back on the amount of butter called for in a recipe (or completely eliminate it in some cases). For example, if you make a box of a flavored rice mix or Stovetop® stuffing, you can completely eliminate the butter/margarine and you would never know the difference. I recently made a salad for a pitch-in dinner that called for 1/2 cup of margarine (eight tablespoons) and I used only two tablespoons instead; everyone still raved about how good it was. Experiment with less butter in your own recipes and you'll be surprised at how little you actually need.

# (29)

**Use less sugar.** Just as with butter and margarine, many recipes will taste just as good with less sugar. In the pitch-in salad I mentioned, I also cut the amount of sugar nearly in half and you would never have known based on the positive feedback it got. Another way to reduce calories in recipes that call for sugar is to substitute at least half of the sugar with a sugar-substitute, such as Splenda® or Equal®. I prefer Splenda® because it is heat-stable, meaning it won't break down or do strange things when heated. Instead of using 1 cup of sugar to make a gallon of iced tea, you could use 1/2 cup of sugar and 1/2 cup of Splenda®. Basically, cut in half whatever amount you currently use in recipes.

You can also find many products in the grocery store that are labeled "Reduced-Sugar." As long as they are actually lower in calories than the regular version, it's a great way to train your palate to require less sugar.

# (30)

**Try a low-fat frozen entrée for a quick and easy lunch.** My favorites include Smart Ones®, Healthy Choice®, and Lean Cuisine®. These meals tend to be moderate in fat, calories, and sodium and are much healthier options than the regular frozen meals. If you don't have time to prepare a lunch to take to work, these are a good alternative to fast food. Many of them won't be enough to fill you up, so you may want to add one or two healthy sides, such as a tossed salad with light dressing, low-fat yogurt, low-fat pudding, a granola bar, or fruit.

# (31)

**Chew sugar-free gum between meals.** This may seem silly, but it's actually pretty effective. Gum keeps your mouth busy so that you are less likely to snack between meals. You may also want to chew gum while you cook or bake if you tend to nibble too much. If you often snack while watching TV or sitting at the computer, try chewing gum instead. Be careful not to chew too many pieces in one day, however, because sugar-free gums and candies can cause gastrointestinal discomfort.

# (32)

**Control portions when dining out.** When the server brings out your meal, immediately cut half or one third of it away with the intention of taking it home as leftovers. Try asking your server to bring out a box out at the beginning of your meal. This way, you're less likely to overeat since the food isn't staring you in the face. Another way to control portions is to share a meal with someone—it saves money too. You may also be able to order from the Kid's Menu if the restaurant will allow it.

The most important thing you can do is listen to your body and stop when you're full. Don't push past fullness just because it tastes good or you don't want to waste it. If you're concerned about the cost of letting food go to waste, remember that trimming your waist line down will likely reduce your healthcare costs in the long-run.

# (33)

**Rarely order appetizers or desserts when dining out.** Unless you have good self-control and are willing to only have a few bites, you will add many unnecessary calories to your meal. One way to ensure you only get a few bites is to split an appetizer or dessert with several other people. Pick one of your favorite restaurants, go to its website and check out the calories in their appetizers and desserts; you may be shocked. If I've saved room for dessert, I'll occasionally order one of my favorites: the "Brownie Bite" from Applebees®. It's a great way to have dessert in moderation since it's only a few bites worth.

# (34)

**Take the edge off your hunger before dining out.** If you're pretty hungry prior to eating out, grab a few pretzels, crackers, or nuts, a piece of fruit, or a slice of cheese before leaving home. This will take the edge off your hunger and help prevent overeating at the restaurant. The calories in a few crackers are much less than the calories you'll consume if you overeat on restaurant food. Another option is to drink a glass of water or diet beverage (e.g., Crystal Light®) in order to take up some room in your stomach.

## (35)

**Go easy on the bread when dining out.** If you normally eat the bread served prior to the entrée, limit yourself to one small piece. If you have a light snack before leaving the house, you won't be facing it on an empty stomach and tempted to eat two or more pieces. You could also save the bread until after your meal and eat in place of a dessert, especially if the bread is a sweet, yeast roll. If you feel that you just cannot wait until the end, you could eat half of a piece prior to the meal and save the other half for the end if you still have room. Don't add much butter, if any, to the bread as it has probably already been brushed with it.

## (36)

**Dip your fork into your salad dressing.** Instead of pouring all of the dressing on top of the salad and making a salad soup, ask that the dressing be brought on the side. Dip your fork into the dressing and then skewer a bite of salad. This way, you'll get to taste the dressing on each bite, but you'll use much less dressing and will save quite a few calories. You'll be amazed at how much dressing is left in the cup once you finish your salad. Also, be sure to eat all of your side salad before the meal because it will take up room in your stomach and you'll have less room for the higher calorie dinner. An added bonus is that you get the health benefits of the veggies.

## (37)

**Choose low-fat sides when dining out.** Instead of always choosing the deep-fried sides, such as French fries and onion rings, try steamed vegetables, a side salad with low-fat dressing, a baked potato (with low-fat toppings), a cup of vegetable soup, green beans, steamed rice, fruit, and so on. If you do order a fried item, such as French fries, get some to share or only eat part of them.

## (38)

**Rarely choose fried entrées.** Instead, choose grilled meat, fish, or poultry. See Tip #18 for examples of lean options. If the meat or poultry has visible fat or skin, be sure to cut or pull it off. Look for a symbol on the menu indicating lower calorie items or check the restaurant's website ahead of time for nutrition information.

## (39)

**When ordering pizza, choose thin crust and low-fat toppings.** Order your pizza with light cheese, or half the amount they normally use. Add as many vegetables as you like and if you prefer meat on your pizza, choose ham or Canadian bacon instead of high-fat ones, such as sausage and pepperoni. If you get breadsticks, limit yourself to one and dip it in tomato sauce rather than garlic butter or cheese sauce. Add a side salad with low-fat dressing so that you won't have as much room for pizza and breadsticks.

Another way to have a lower calorie pizza is to make your own with part-skim mozzarella cheese, vegetables, and turkey pepperoni, Canadian bacon, or reduced-fat sausage (Jimmy Dean® has a 50% less fat option). I often use whole wheat pocketless pita bread as a quick and easy crust. For the sauce I either use a ready-made version or I'll put diced Italian tomatoes in my food processor and add some minced garlic. In order to pack more nutrients into your sauce, process other vegetables along with the tomatoes and garlic, such as zucchini, spinach, mushrooms, onions, and green peppers. This way, you're able to sneak in more veggies without anyone knowing (this works great for picky kiddos; they'll never know).

## (40)

**Avoid high-fat toppings on your sandwiches.** These include creamy sauces, such as Ranch and mayonnaise (unless they offer light mayo), bacon, and cheese. If the sandwich you order comes with one of these toppings, then simply ask that it be left off. Instead, top your sandwich with lettuce, tomato, pickles, onion, ketchup, mustard, barbecue sauce, and so on.

## (41)

**Avoid large or super-sized items at fast food restaurants.** In general, you should try to limit fast food to once per week or so (unless you are willing to order healthier items). If you do eat fast food, choose lower calorie items, such as a grilled chicken sandwich or wrap, a grilled chicken salad with a light dressing, chicken nuggets, a single burger with a side salad, fruit, and/or yogurt, or a bean burrito. Many fast food restaurants now offer fruit as a side, such as mandarin oranges, apples, and mixed fruit.

If you get French fries, stick to a small order or share a medium with a friend. Many times, when my family and I eat out, we'll get a side of fruit or veggies with our meal and then split an order of fries. One of my favorite fast food restaurants is Chick-Fil-A®. They use whole chicken breasts rather than a processed version, they cook their food in peanut oil, which is a heart-healthy unsaturated fat, and they offer fresh fruits and veggies. Plus, there are several meal combinations that fit into a calorie counter's budget, not to mention their tasty Icedream® dessert, which is made from skim milk. A small Icedream® cone only has 160 calories.

For a while, ask for a Nutrition Guide at each restaurant you normally eat and use it to find the lower calorie items. For most women, try to limit the calories in your meal to 700 or less and for men, 800 or less. This may seem tedious and time-consuming at first, but it's a great way to become familiar with what foods are highest in calories and before long, you'll be a pro at sorting through menus.

# (42)

**At Mexican restaurants, avoid fried items and high-fat toppings.** If you aren't sure whether or not an item is fried, ask your server. High-fat toppings include sour cream, cheese sauces, and guacamole. As a side dish, order a salad with low-fat dressing, rice, or beans. Order your dish with extra lettuce and add salsa for more veggies. If you like to eat the tortilla chips prior to the entrée (who doesn't?), limit yourself to just enough to take the edge off your hunger and dip them in salsa rather than a cheese sauce. In general, choose chicken or beans instead of beef for the entrée. At Taco Bell I always substitute beans for meat, and ask that the sour cream be left off just to make it a bit healthier.

# (43)

**At Italian restaurants, avoid dishes with creamy sauces.** This includes Alfredo-type and cheese-laden dishes. Find the menu online and look for the nutrition information so that you can choose a lower calorie/fat option. You can also ask that the cheese be left off the top of the dish in order to save some calories. There have also been times when I ordered a dish and asked that a marinara or tomato sauce be substituted for the creamy one it normally came with. In general, some lower calorie options include minestrone and pasta fagioli soups as well as spaghetti marinara. Have salad prior to the meal (with the dressing on the side) to help take up some room in your stomach and limit bread to one piece. The most important thing to remember no matter what you order is to stop when you're full.

# (44)

**At Chinese restaurants, limit breaded/fried items.** Choose grilled or stir-fried meats without breading, steamed rice (brown rice if available), and clear soups. Find meals that include vegetables or order a side of steamed veggies. Also try to go easy on the soy sauce since it's loaded in sodium.

# (45)

**Beware of buffets.** For the most part, try to avoid them altogether. It's too hard for most people to eat an appropriate amount of food because you feel like you need to eat your money's worth. If you do find yourself at a buffet, be sure to start with a salad to take up some room in your stomach. Then, be sure to balance your plate with both starchy and non-starchy veggies, a lean protein, and fruit. Save room for only a few bites of dessert rather than a full portion. And, most importantly, stop eating before you become uncomfortably full.

## (46)

**Choose lower-fat options when dining out for breakfast.** Examples include omelets made with egg whites (or Egg Beaters®), Canadian bacon or lean ham, oatmeal, grits, yogurt, English muffins, bran muffins, or whole wheat toast without butter, fresh fruit, pancakes with light syrup or only a small amount of regular syrup, and skim milk. In general, try to avoid high-fat items, such as biscuits, croissants, danishes, donuts, pastries, sweet rolls, bacon, sausage, gravy, and stuffed French toast. Again, it might be helpful to go to the restaurant's website first in order to find the lower calorie items.

Of course, it's fine to have a "treat" breakfast occasionally, but remember to only eat until you're full and then watch your calorie intake a bit closer for lunch and dinner.

One of my favorite breakfast treats is biscuits and gravy and every now and then I give into a craving. In order to save calories, I get the gravy on the side and spoon just enough over the biscuit to taste it on every bite without drenching it. Better yet, I make my own at home. Here's a lower-fat recipe for you (no extra charge!). Take 1/3 of a roll of Jimmy Dean® 50% less fat sausage and brown it in a skillet (or brown the entire roll and put 2/3 of it in the freezer to use on a homemade pizza). There's hardly any grease to make the gravy, so you'll need to add 2–3 tablespoons of oil (preferably canola or olive).

Next, sprinkle 3 tablespoons of flour over the sausage/oil mixture and whisk until absorbed. Add approximately 3 cups of skim milk and whisk until smooth. Season with a small pinch of nutmeg, and salt and pepper to taste. Simmer until thickened. Serve over biscuits made from Reduced-Fat Bisquick® alongside some fresh fruit. Yum! You can even serve this to your overnight guests and they'll never know it's lower in fat.

# (47)

**Stick to small sizes at ice cream restaurants (e.g., Dairy Queen® or Baskin Robbins®).** Lower calorie options include a small ice cream cone, a small sundae, an ice cream sandwich, a Dilly® Bar (Dairy Queen®), a StarKiss® (Dairy Queen®), a fudge bar, low-fat or non-fat frozen yogurt, and no-sugar-added products. One way to help fit it in the calories of an ice cream treat is to eat a light meal for dinner. Don't be tempted to skip a meal to save up calories. Then, you'll want to eat a much larger portion because you'll be so hungry. If this helps you, remember that a small candy bar Blizzard® from Dairy Queen® has approximately 500-700 calories (that's about a third or more of what most women need in an entire day)!

# (48)

**Limit movie popcorn.** As you can probably imagine, movie popcorn is high in both calories and fat since most theaters pop it in coconut oil. Unfortunately, coconut oil is high in saturated fat (the kind that clogs arteries). Here are some fun facts: the average medium, buttered bag of popcorn contains a whopping 1170 calories and 90 grams of fat. A medium, unbuttered bag contains 900 calories and 60 grams of fat, and a small, unbuttered bag contains 400 calories and 27 grams of fat.

If you really want some, choose the small, unbuttered bag or share a medium with a friend. One way to help balance out the calories is to have a light meal earlier or later in the day (depending on the time of the movie). You could also do extra physical activity to help spend the additional calories. Make sure to avoid the temptation of a free refill and choose a low-calorie beverage to go with it (e.g., diet soda or water). In order to help curb your craving, plan to go to a movie that is soon after you've eaten lunch or dinner so that you won't be facing your temptation on an empty stomach.

## (49)

**Include sweet treats as part of your meal.** In order to allow yourself treats in moderation, leave a little room at the end of dinner. This way, you're not eating the treat to fill you up when you're hungry, which means you'll eat less of it. This allows you to taste the treat and satisfy your sweet-tooth without overdoing it. I like to keep peanut M&M's® in the cabinet because I can grab about 10 after dinner as a treat. I don't actually count them out, but I figured you might wonder about how many I eat at a time. Other options include a couple of small cookies, one medium-sized cookie, a few Hershey's kisses, two mini candy bars, three bite-sized candy bars, and so on. If you like dark chocolate, it's a good choice since it contains antioxidants (disease fighters).

# (50)

**If you have a craving for chocolate milk, make your own.** Use skim milk and add sugar-free chocolate syrup for fewer calories than the commercially prepared version. Another option, that I often do, is to choose the commercially prepared chocolate milk and dilute it with skim milk. Have it with a meal, as your afternoon snack, or as part of your evening snack. Limit yourself to one glass (8–12 ounces).

This may seem like an insignificant tip to include, but I did so to demonstrate how I compromise or make small changes in my diet to save calories. Hopefully you'll apply a similar strategy in all areas of your diet in order to cut calories here and there. It's these types of small changes that result in big changes over time. Plus, it's this type of compromise that makes a healthier diet easier to maintain over the long-term.

# (51)

**Choose foods based on what your body needs rather than only what sounds good.** I believe that food should be enjoyable, and believe me, I enjoy food. However, it's also important to consider the fact that your body needs a certain amount of nutrients in order to work properly. If you only eat what sounds good without any consideration of nutrient content, your body probably isn't getting all the nutrients it needs. For example, when choosing a snack, consider what food group is lacking from your diet for the day. If you haven't had any fruit yet, then choose fruit, or if you haven't had enough calcium, then choose yogurt, cheese, or milk. If you haven't had many veggies for the day, then have a nice, big salad for dinner.

A healthy diet is a balancing act. When planning dinner, try to have a balanced plate with both starchy and non-starchy vegetables, a whole grain of some sort (e.g., pasta, tortilla, or rice), a small portion of lean meat, and fruit. Remember to have variety, balance, and moderation in your diet.

## (52)

**Limit your sodium (or salt) intake.** Choose and prepare foods with less salt because a high salt intake is linked to high blood pressure. If you're accustomed to eating salty foods, then just retrain your taste buds. Limit your use of the salt shaker and try using other ways to add flavor to your foods, such as herbs and spices, salt-free seasoning blends, onion, garlic, and lemon juice. Also watch out for foods that are already high in salt, including pickles, olives, soy sauce, lunchmeats, convenience foods like boxed or frozen meals and side dishes, canned soups and sauces. As you begin to reduce your salt intake, your taste buds will adjust and they won't "need" as much as they used to.

It's recommended to limit sodium intake to 2300 milligrams (mg) a day, which divided by three meals is about 700 mg per meal (with some left for snacks). Think of that number when looking at the labels of frozen meals and soups. When grocery shopping, look for items that are labeled "reduced-sodium," "sodium-free," or "low sodium." By the way, a food that contains 140 mg of sodium or less per serving is considered "low sodium."

Eating more fruits, fresh or frozen vegetables, fresh lean meats as opposed to processed meats, and whole grains can help to reduce your sodium intake because they're naturally low in sodium. Keep in mind that eating more of what you should leaves less room for what you shouldn't.

## (53)

**Limit high-calorie coffee drinks.** A large mocha, hot chocolate, latte, or Frappuccino® made with whole milk can pack 400–500 calories. Instead, opt for the small size and have it made "light" (or at least with non-fat milk). Also, skip the whipped cream on top. These changes will cut the calorie content in half, but you'll still want to count the drink as your snack or in place of other sweets.

## (54)

**Don't eat out of boredom.** It's common in our country to eat because you just want something to do and because it's enjoyable. If this is the case for you, find other activities you enjoy (e.g., volunteer work, dance class, aerobics, knitting, scrapbooking, playing a sport, working in the yard, painting, writing, reading, woodworking, pottery) Keep yourself busy so that you have less time to think about food. Put a list of ideas on the pantry door so that when you're tempted to eat when you're not actually hungry, you can see some other ideas.

## (55)

**If you eat when you're sad or mad, find other ways to comfort yourself.** Instead of cheering yourself up with comfort food, call a friend or relative, listen to music, read a book, or exercise. A great way to release anger is to exercise, especially with kickboxing, a punching bag, walking, or jogging.

Emotional eating and food addictions are quite common in the United States. If you have trouble breaking these habits on your own, you may benefit from making an appointment with a behavioral therapist, pastor, or counselor for more advice on dealing with anger, sadness, or depression in a healthy way.

## (56)

**Subscribe to a healthy cooking magazine or buy low-fat cookbooks.** This is a great way to learn more about how to cook with less fat. A couple of my favorite magazines are *Light and Tasty* and *Cooking Light*. Go to your local super market or bookstore in order to buy a trial copy before you decide to subscribe to one of them. For quick, healthy meal ideas, check out the book "Quick Fix Meals" by Robin Miller (she has a show on the Food Network as well).

## (57)

**Practice self-control.** If you've mastered all of the previous tips, then you are following a pretty healthy diet, which means you have made some wonderful changes in your life that will help you achieve a healthier body. Even though you've learned which foods are healthier, it's still important to eat them in moderation. It's great to learn to make better food choices, but it's just as important to **know when to stop**. You were created to know when you're hungry and when you're full, so pay attention and follow your body's lead. Eat when you're hungry (on a regular schedule) and stop when you're full.

# (58)

**Don't give up!** When you mess up and eat more than you should, don't let it keep you from getting back up and trying again. We all eat more than we should sometimes or choose foods that aren't the healthiest, but there's always tomorrow and you can try again. I'm sure in the past when you've tried a fad diet, you have messed up or eaten something you weren't supposed to and just said "Forget it!". There's no need to do that when you're simply learning to eat healthier. Just realize your blunder and try to eat better at your next meal; simple as that! Also remember that it may take a while for you to reach a healthy weight, but stick with these tips and you will get there—don't give up!

# *Wrap-up*

You made it! Hopefully, you've found this book helpful and will continue to find it helpful along your journey to healthier eating and/or weight loss. Remember to keep following the tips because it takes time and commitment to reach and maintain a healthy weight. You may need to go back through the tips to see if there are any you could follow more closely in order to cut a few more calories. Be sure to check out the tools I've provided in the Resources section to help you along the way. There's also a list of the tips at the end of the Resources that might serve as a handy reference. Be sure to sign up for my free electronic newsletter on my website at booksbyapril.com. Good luck to you and remember to never give up! A healthy weight is coming your way.

If you are serious about weight loss, I highly recommend that you see an RD (Registered Dietitian) in your area. If your insurance company requires a referral, talk to your Primary Care Physician about your desire to meet with a dietitian for weight loss. Your doctor should have no problem giving you a referral since maintaining a healthy weight is so vital to your overall health. An RD can give you an individualized meal plan based on your food preferences and calorie needs and can provide ongoing moral support throughout your journey. One way to find an RD in your area is to visit the American Dietetics Association's website at eatright.org.

# *Resources*

BACK TO BASICS

# Food Pyramid

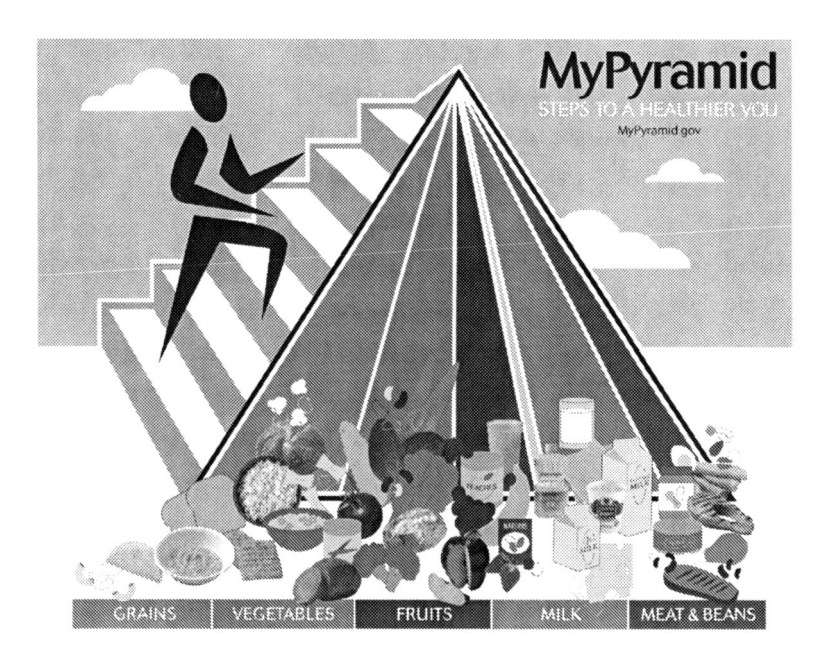

Source: mypyramid.gov

# Sample Meal Pattern

Here is a sample meal pattern if you are the type of person who prefers a more structured guide. Keep in mind that **this is only a guide** and is not meant to meet everyone's individual calorie needs. It should also be noted that this pattern is flexible and can be adjusted based on your eating preferences. For example, if you'd rather not have a serving from the milk group with lunch, then have it as an afternoon snack between lunch and dinner or swap it out for a different food group from another meal. The amount of food suggested below are minimums for most people, so add more servings as your body leads you—just eat until you're full. Remember, if you get hungry between meals during the day refer to Tip #9 for healthy snack ideas.

## Step 1

Use the patterns provided in the following table as a guide for making choices in Step 2.

| Breakfast | Lunch | Dinner | Evening Snack |
|---|---|---|---|
| 1–2 grains<br>1 milk<br>1 fruit | 2 grains<br>2–3 oz. protein<br>1 fruit and/or vegetable<br>1 milk | 1–2 grains<br>3 oz. protein<br>2–3 vegetables<br>1 fruit | 1–2 grains<br>1 milk |

## Step 2

Select choices from the categories below according to the pattern in Step 1.

| Category | Choices | |
|---|---|---|
| *Grains* <br> *5–8 serv/day* | 1 slice whole wheat bread <br> 1 cup dry cereal <br> 1/2 cup cooked cereal <br> 1/2 whole wheat bagel <br> 1/2 English muffin <br> Small dinner roll or muffin | 1/2 cup brown rice <br> 1/2 cup whole wheat pasta <br> 3 cups popcorn <br> 6 soda crackers <br> 3 graham cracker squares <br> 1 tortilla |
| *Milk* <br> *3 serv/day* | 1 cup skim or 1% milk <br> 1 cup low-fat yogurt <br> 2 slices or 1/3 cup shredded cheese | |
| *Fruits* <br> *3–4 serv/day* | 1/2 cup chopped fresh <br> 1/2 cup canned (light) <br> Small piece whole fresh <br> 1/2 cup berries | 1/2 grapefruit <br> 16 grapes <br> 1/4 cup dried <br> 1/2 cup 100% juice (4 oz.) |

| Category | Choices | |
|---|---|---|
| Vegetables 4–6 serv/day | 1/2 cup cooked<br>1/2 cup raw chopped<br>6 baby carrots<br>1 cup raw leafy<br>1/2 cup juice (4 oz.) | Starchy: corn, peas, beans, potatoes<br>Non-starchy: broccoli, carrots, onions, Brussels sprouts, tomatoes, cucumbers, greens, cabbage, green beans, lettuce, asparagus, cauliflower, peppers |
| Meat/Proteins* 5–6 oz./day | 1 oz. lean meat, fish, or poultry<br>Note: see Tip #18 for examples of lean meats<br><br>1 oz. cheese<br>1/4 cup low-fat cottage cheese | 1 egg or 1/4 cup egg substitute<br>1/4 cup tofu<br>1/4 cup beans<br>1/2 oz. nuts or seeds<br>1 Tbsp peanut butter<br>1/4 cup canned tuna or salmon (water-packed) |

*Note: 1 oz. cheese, 1/4 cup cottage cheese, 1/4 cup canned tuna or salmon, 1 egg, 1/4 cup egg substitute, 1 oz. tofu, 1/4 cup beans, and 1 Tbsp. peanut butter are all equivalent to 1 oz. meat, fish, or poultry.

# Sample Food Record Evaluation

Here is a sample food record evaluation that shows how to break down your current diet into the different food groups. Below the evaluation is a discussion of what is shown. I encourage you to keep a record of everything you eat for a few days in order to get an idea of how your diet compares to the recommended amounts. A food record helps you determine what you need to eat more or less of in order to better meet your nutrient needs and to find out where unnecessary calories may be lurking.

| Meal | How it Breaks Down |
|---|---|
| **Breakfast**<br>1 cup Raisin Bran<br>1 cup milk | **Breakfast**<br>1 grain<br>1 milk |
| **Lunch**<br>Ham sandwich (2 oz. ham)<br>Lettuce, tomato (1 cup total)<br>1 serving of Wheat Thins®<br>1 medium-sized apple | **Lunch**<br>2 oz. protein, 2 grains<br>1 vegetable<br>1 grain<br>2 fruits |
| **Dinner**<br>6 oz. chicken breast<br>1 medium-sized baked potato<br>1/2 cup macaroni and cheese<br>1 small dinner roll<br>2 Oreos® | **Dinner**<br>6 oz. protein<br>2 vegetables<br>1 grain<br>1 grain<br>Discretionary calories |
| **Snack**<br>1 cup of potato chips | **Snack**<br>Discretionary calories |

| **Actual Totals** | **Recommended Totals** |
|---|---|
| 6 grains | 5-8 grains |
| 1 milk | 3 milks |
| 8 oz. protein | 5-6 oz. protein |
| 3 vegetables | 4-6 vegetables |
| 2 fruits | 3-4 fruits |

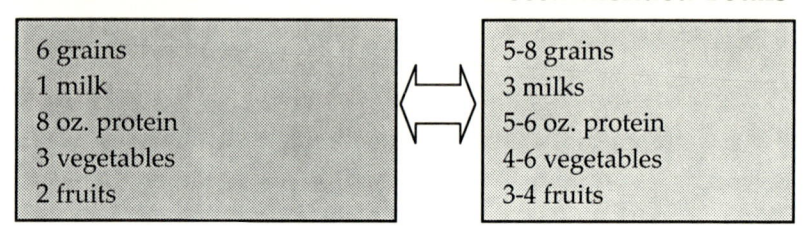

## *Discussion*

If you compare the total intake to the recommended amounts, you will find that this diet is adequate in grains and protein (actually, a little heavy on protein); however, the diet is lacking in milk and other calcium-rich foods, vegetables, and fruit, which is quite typical of the American diet.

In order to change this diet to better meet nutrient needs, I would suggest adding a fruit serving at breakfast and/or dinner, adding cheese to the ham sandwich or a side of yogurt at lunch for the milk group, substitute a non-starchy vegetable for one of the grains at dinner, and reduce the chicken breast to a three- or four-ounce portion. I would also suggest a more nutrient-rich snack as well, such as cereal with skim milk or low-fat pudding with a few vanilla wafers (in order to get that last serving of milk in).

## Sample Menus

I get asked quite often for sample menus and I normally hesitate to give them out because I would rather you learn how to design a healthy meal yourself based on the information I've given you throughout the book. Also, we all have unique calorie needs based on our age, sex, weight, height, body composition, and activity level, so one set of sample menus won't fit the needs of everyone. However, I decided to at least give you a glimpse of what I might eat in an average week and then let you tweak them as needed to fit your individual needs.

These menus should serve as a guide to help you learn healthy combinations; **they are not meant for you to follow exactly.** I want you to see how I fit all foods into my diet in moderation. You will notice that some foods are not the healthiest, and that's okay because they don't displace healthy foods, meaning that they aren't keeping me from meeting my nutrient needs with vegetables, proteins, dairy, and whole grains. As you know by now, I believe that a diet that includes small amounts of treats on a regular basis is much easier to stick to than a restrictive diet in which you avoid them.

If you want to try and use these meals as a guide, that's fine, but realize that you may need to eat a little more or a little less depending on your calorie needs— follow your body's lead. For example, if you are a male these meals will likely not be enough food for you, so follow the meal pattern, but increase the serving sizes so that you get full, but not stuffed. On the other hand, if you are a small-framed female over the age of 50, these meals may be too large for you, so don't force yourself to eat past fullness in order to fit it all in; stop when you're full.

If you don't like a food that I've listed, feel free to substitute something else in its place, but try to make it something that is in the same food group and similar in caloric content. For example, if I have green beans listed as a side dish and you don't like them, substitute a vegetable you do like, such as carrots. Or if I have Raisin Bran listed for breakfast and you don't like it, then choose a different high-fiber cereal instead. Again, I just want you to get an idea of what a healthy, balanced diet looks like.

Also, you'll notice that I've included times to give you an idea about how to space your meals throughout the day. Small deviations are fine, but try to shoot for 4–6 hours between meals (see Tip #1 for more details). Lastly, I've included an afternoon snack in case you get hungry between lunch and dinner. Don't feel obligated to fit it in if you're not hungry, but if you do, remember to only eat enough to hold you until dinner.

## Day 1

| | |
|---|---|
| *Breakfast* 8:00am | 1/2 cup Fiber One with Honey Clusters® cereal + 2/3 cup Cinnamon Toast Crunch® <br> 1 cup skim milk <br> 1/2 banana |
| *Lunch* 12:00pm | 2 slices whole wheat bread <br> Lean turkey or ham (2 oz.) <br> 1 Tbsp. light mayo or Miracle Whip® <br> 1 slice of cheese <br> Lettuce and/or Tomato <br> 1 serving of Lays Natural Reduced-Fat Potato Chips® <br> 1/2 medium sliced apple <br> A few M&M's® (8–10) <br> Water or low-calorie beverage (see Tip #6 for ideas) |
| *Snack* 4:00pm | 1 serving of Honey-Wheat pretzel twists (refer to package for serving size) <br> Low-calorie beverage |
| *Dinner* 6:00pm | 1 cup whole wheat pasta (Barilla® brand) <br> 1/2 cup tomato sauce with sautéed zucchini and yellow squash added <br> 3 oz. skinless chicken breast <br> 1 1/2 cups tossed salad with 2 Tbsp. reduced-fat salad dressing <br> 1 slice light garlic bread <br> 2 Oreo® cookies <br> Water or low-calorie beverage |
| *Snack* 9:30pm | 1 1/2 cups dry cereal of your choice, such as Honey Nut Cheerios® <br> 1 cup skim milk |

## Day 2

| | |
|---|---|
| *Breakfast* 8:00am | 1 medium whole wheat bagel<br>2 Tbsp. reduced-sugar jelly or light cream cheese<br>6–8 oz. calcium-fortified orange juice |
| *Lunch* 12:00pm | 2 cups tossed salad with reduced-fat salad dressing<br>2 oz. skinless chicken breast chunks (in salad)<br>1/2 cup fruit (canned or fresh chopped)<br>1/2 cup low-fat cottage cheese<br>1 chocolate Rice Krispies Treats® bar<br>Water or low-calorie beverage |
| *Snack* 4:00pm | 10–20 medium-sized grapes and low-calorie beverage |
| *Dinner* 6:00pm | 1 cup brown rice<br>1 cup stir-fry veggies (e.g., broccoli, carrots, snow peas, water chestnuts, red peppers, onion) in sauce<br>3 oz. skinless chicken breast or lean sirloin<br>1/2 cup fresh fruit salad (e.g., pineapple, mandarin oranges, grapes, strawberries)<br>2-3 pieces Dove® dark chocolate<br>Water or low-calorie beverage |
| *Snack* 9:30pm | 1 slice cheddar or Colby-Jack cheese<br>1 serving of Triscuits® or other crackers, baked chips, or Natural Lay's®<br>Water or low-calorie beverage |

## Day 3

| | |
|---|---|
| Breakfast<br>7:30am | 1 cup Maple Brown Sugar Mini-Wheats®<br>1 cup skim milk<br>1/2 cup sliced strawberries |
| Lunch<br>11:30pm | Lean Cuisine® or Smart Ones® frozen entrée<br>1/2 cup fresh pineapple or 1 kiwi<br>1 pudding cup<br>Water or low-calorie beverage |
| Snack<br>4:00pm | Palmful of mixed nuts |
| Dinner<br>6:00pm | 1 whole wheat tortilla<br>Filling: beans, salsa, 2% milk shredded cheddar cheese, extra lean ground beef seasoned (optional; could leave beef out and make this your meatless meal)<br>Topping: shredded lettuce (green leafy and iceberg), green peppers, and shredded carrots, light sour cream and more salsa<br>1/2 cup red beans and rice (e.g., Zatarain's®)<br>1/2 cup canned light pears<br>1–2 small chocolate chip cookies<br>Water or low-calorie beverage |
| Snack<br>10:00 pm | 6-8 crackers with a total of two tablespoons of peanut butter spread over them or a package of Reduced-Fat peanut butter and cheese cracker sandwiches<br>1 cup chocolate milk (mixed with skim milk) |

| Day 4 | |
|---|---|
| Breakfast 8:00am | 1/2 cup Fiber One® with Honey Clusters cereal + 2/3 cup Honey Nut Cheerios® 1 cup skim milk 1/2 cup orange juice or 1/2 banana |
| Lunch 12:00pm | 2 slices whole wheat bread 2 Tbsp. peanut butter 1 Tbsp. low-sugar jelly 6 oz. low-fat yogurt 1/2–1 serving of Multigrain Tostitos® (tortilla chips) Water or low-calorie beverage |
| Snack 4:00pm | Chocolate chip granola bar (low-fat) Water or low-calorie beverage |
| Dinner 6:00pm | 3 oz. meatloaf (made with extra lean ground beef) 1/2 cup mashed potatoes (made with skim milk and trans fat-free margarine) 1/2 cup steamed carrots 1 cup spinach salad with chopped pears, dried cranberries, and light vinaigrette Palmful of Raisinettes® Water or low-calorie beverage |
| Snack 9:30pm | 1–2 slices whole grain cinnamon raisin bread or a bagel 1 cup skim milk |

# BACK TO BASICS

## Day 5

| | |
|---|---|
| *Breakfast* 7:30am | 2 small whole wheat waffles (e.g., Go Lean® brand) 2 Tbsp. pancake syrup (use "light" if you use a larger quantity) 1/4 cup berries on top 1 cup skim milk |
| *Lunch* 11:30am | 1-2 cups vegetable soup Grilled cheese (made with whole wheat bread and 2% milk cheese) 1/2 to 1 medium fresh pear Water or low-calorie beverage |
| *Snack* 3:30pm | 1 serving of Whole-grain Goldfish® crackers Water or low-calorie beverage |
| *Dinner* 6:30pm | Tuna salad on whole wheat bread (only use half of yolks and light mayo) 1 serving of baked French Fries 1/2 cup mixed vegetables cooked in chicken or vegetable stock/broth 1/2 cup mandarin oranges Chocolate graham crackers (one sheet) Water or low-calorie beverage |
| *Snack* 9:30pm | Ice cream cone with reduced-fat ice cream (e.g., Edy's Slow Churned®) |

## Day 6

| | |
|---|---|
| *Breakfast* 8:00am | 1 Jimmy Dean D-Lights® breakfast sandwich or make your own with a whole wheat English muffin, 2 egg whites cooked, 1 slice Canadian bacon or a turkey sausage patty, and 1 slice 2% milk cheese<br>1 cup calcium-fortified o.j. |
| *Lunch* 12:00pm | Bagel pizza (made with whole wheat bagel, turkey pepperoni, part-skim mozzarella, sauce, and veggies of choice)<br>Baby carrots with light Ranch dressing<br>1/2 cup grapes<br>Water or low-calorie beverage |
| *Snack* 4:00pm | 1 banana |
| *Dinner* 6:00pm | 3–4 skinless chicken tenders marinated in Italian dressing and baked<br>Steamed broccoli/cauliflower/carrot mix<br>1/2 cup whole wheat noodles boiled in chicken broth<br>1/2 cup fruit salad (kiwi, banana, grapes, pineapple)<br>3–5 vanilla wafers<br>Water or low-calorie beverage |
| *Snack* 10:00pm | 1 snack-size bag of microwave popcorn (100 calorie pack Kettle Corn)<br>1/2 palmful of peanut M&M's<br>Water or low-calorie beverage |

## Day 7

| | |
|---|---|
| *Breakfast* 9:00am | 2 slices whole wheat toast with 2 tsp. trans fat-free margarine and low sugar jelly<br>Scrambled eggs (1 whole egg + 2 egg whites cooked in non-stick spray)<br>1 oz. Canadian bacon or 2 slices turkey bacon<br>6–8 oz. calcium-fortified orange juice |
| *Lunch* 1:00pm | 1 Morningstar Farms® veggie corndog (try it, it's better than you expect)<br>1 cup low-fat yogurt<br>1 fruit cup<br>1 Nabisco® 100-Calorie Pack dessert<br>Water or low-calorie beverage |
| *Snack* 4:00pm | One serving of Multigrain Tostitos® (tortilla chips) |
| *Dinner* 7:00pm | 3 oz. pork loin (trimmed of fat and cooked in slow cooker)<br>1/2 cup green beans<br>1 cob of corn (with spray butter)<br>Sliced fresh cucumber and tomato with light Ranch dressing<br>1 whole wheat dinner roll with 1 tsp. honey<br>Water or low-calorie beverage |
| *Snack* 10:00pm | 1 packet of oatmeal<br>1 cup skim milk |

# Sample Grocery List

I have provided a sample grocery to give you an idea of how to plan a week's worth of meals. To generate my grocery lists, I first make a list of dinners for the week and then begin building the list based on the food that is needed for those dinners. Next, I think of breakfast, lunch, and snack foods needed for the week and add those to the list. I like to group my foods and put them in the order of the store so that it's quicker once I get there.

**Dinner menus for the week**
1. Pork chops, baked potatoes, carrots, and fruit salad
2. Cheese ravioli with tomato sauce, tossed salad, and garlic bread
3. Chicken stir-fry with brown rice and pear slices
4. Meatloaf, sweet potatoes, green beans, and fruit cocktail
5. Chicken and black bean burritos, red beans & rice, strawberries

## Produce
- ☐ Potatoes
- ☐ Sweet potatoes
- ☐ Baby carrots
- ☐ Apples, strawberries, and kiwi
- ☐ Pears
- ☐ Bananas (for breakfast and/or lunch)
- ☐ Bag of Romaine salad (chop some for top of burritos)
- ☐ Tomatoes, cucumber, and green pepper (to add to salad)
- ☐ Bag of stir-fry veggie blend (some bags contain sauce as well for making stir-fry; could also find in frozen section).

## Meat/Dairy
- ☐ Lean pork loin chops
- ☐ Boneless, skinless chicken breasts or tenderloins
- ☐ 1 lb. extra lean (4% fat) or lean (8% fat) ground beef
- ☐ Lean ham from deli (for lunch)
- ☐ Sliced Colby-jack or 2% milk cheese slices (for lunch)
- ☐ Skim milk (for adults) and whole milk (for toddlers age 1–2)
- ☐ Light or low-fat yogurt (for lunch and/or snack)
- ☐ Light sour cream
- ☐ Eggs (for meatloaf and/or breakfast)

## Canned Items
- ☐ Light Fruit cocktail
- ☐ Green beans
- ☐ Pasta sauce (chunky garden combination for more veggies)
- ☐ Diced Italian tomatoes (for pasta sauce)
- ☐ Salsa (for burritos and an evening snack)
- ☐ Black beans
- ☐ Fruit cups (for lunch)
- ☐ Light salad dressing
- ☐ Low-calorie beverages (e.g., Crystal Lite)
- ☐ 100% fruit juice

## Dry Goods/Boxed Items
- ☐ Loaf of whole wheat bread (for lunch)
- ☐ Brown rice
- ☐ Red beans & rice (e.g., Zatarains®)
- ☐ Taco seasoning
- ☐ Whole wheat tortillas
- ☐ Fiber One® with Honey Clusters (for breakfast)
- ☐ Honey Nut Cheerios® (to mix with Fiber One®)
- ☐ Low-fat granola bars (for lunch and/or snack)
- ☐ Goldfish® crackers (for lunch and/or snack)
- ☐ Multigrain tortilla chips (for lunch and/or snack)
- ☐ Oreos® or other cookie (for dessert after dinner)

## Frozen Items
- ☐ Garlic bread (e.g., Lite Texas Toast)
- ☐ Bag of cheese ravioli
- ☐ Healthy lunches (e.g., Lean Cuisine®, Smart Ones®, Healthy Choice®)
- ☐ Whole wheat waffles (e.g., Kashi Go Lean®)
- ☐ Morningstar Farms® corndogs (for lunch)

## Back to Basics Tip Sheet

1. Eat three regular meals every day.
2. Plan ahead.
3. Stop eating when you're full.
4. Make time for breakfast.
5. Get more fiber.
6. Limit sugary drinks.
7. Have three servings of calcium-rich foods daily.
8. Slow down.
9. Choose healthier snacks.
10. Allow treats in moderation.
11. Eat more vegetables.
12. Eat more fruit.
13. Limit your fat intake.
14. Choose foods that are "light," "low-fat," or "reduced-fat."
15. Use low-fat cooking methods.
16. Trim fat and skin from meat and poultry.
17. Limit high-fat meats.
18. Choose lean meat, fish, and poultry.
19. Eat more legumes.
20. Have a meatless dinner at least once a week.
21. Eat, drink, and cook with low-fat dairy products.
22. Use low-fat or light condiments.
23. Top baked potatoes with low-fat or fat-free toppings.
24. Top pasta with tomato-based sauces.
25. Choose clear soups over creamy ones.
26. Use more egg whites than yolks.
27. Compare calories on the Nutrition Label.
28. Use less butter and/or margarine.
29. Use less sugar.
30. Try a low-fat frozen entrée for a quick and easy lunch.
31. Chew sugar-free gum between meals.
32. Control portions when dining out.

33. Rarely order appetizers or desserts when dining out.
34. Take the edge off your hunger before dining out.
35. Go easy on the bread when dining out.
36. Dip your fork into your salad dressing.
37. Choose low-fat sides when dining out.
38. Rarely choose fried entrees.
39. When ordering pizza, choose thin crust and low-fat toppings.
40. Avoid high-fat toppings on your sandwiches.
41. Avoid large or super-sized items at fast food restaurants.
42. At Mexican restaurants, avoid fried items and high-fat toppings.
43. At Italian restaurants, avoid dishes with creamy sauces.
44. At Chinese restaurants, limit breaded/fried items.
45. Beware of buffets.
46. Choose lower-fat options when dining out for breakfast.
47. Stick to small sizes at ice cream restaurants (e.g., Dairy Queen® or Baskin Robbins®).
48. Limit movie popcorn.
49. Include sweet treats as part of your meal.
50. If you have a craving for chocolate milk, make your own.
51. Choose foods based on what your body needs rather than only what sounds good.
52. Limit your sodium (or salt) intake.
53. Limit high-calorie coffee drinks.
54. Don't eat out of boredom.
55. If you eat when you're sad or mad, find other ways to comfort yourself.
56. Subscribe to a healthy cooking magazine or buy low-fat cookbooks.
57. Practice self-control.
58. Don't give up!

# About the Author

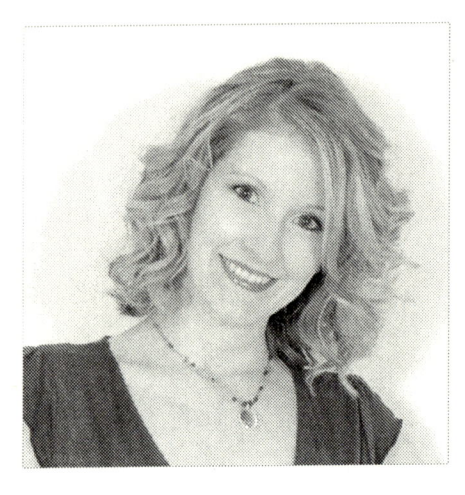

April is a wife and mother of two who resides in Indiana. She enjoys cooking, watching The Food Network, reading magazines and inspiring books, spending time with friends and family, and is an active member of her church.

April received her Bachelor's degree in Dietetics from Indiana University and went on to complete an internship through the IU School of Medicine in Indianapolis (IUPUI). She has worked as a community dietitian and taught nutrition at a community college. She has spent most of her career as a Clinical Dietitian in a hospital, educating on an outpatient basis. Currently, April spends most of her time as a work-at-home mom, as a co-owner of the Indiana Weight Loss and Wellness Institute (indianaweightloss.net) and as owner of Books by April (booksbyapril.com).

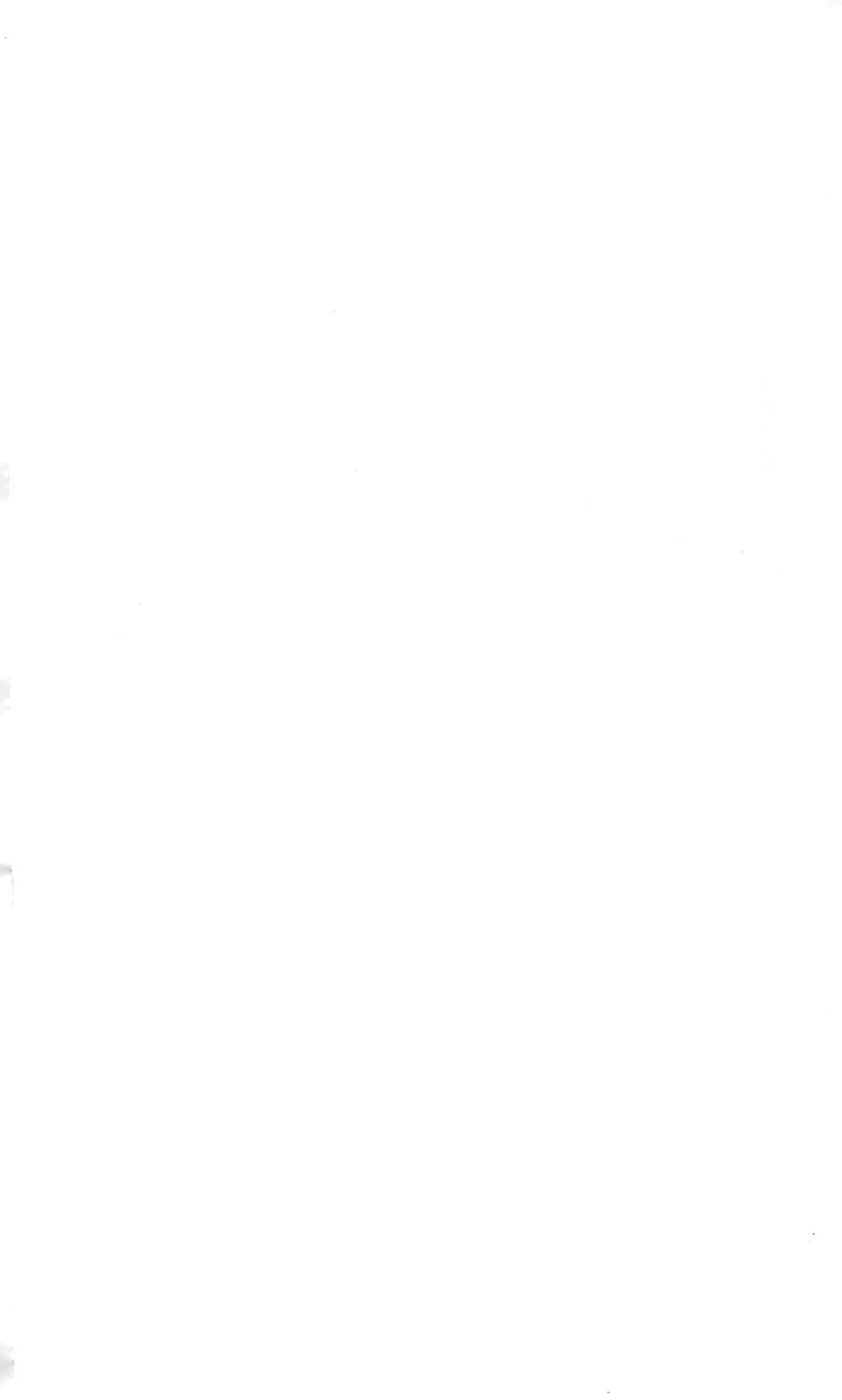

Printed in the United States
217930BV00001B/2/A